Narrative-Based Practice
in Speech-Language Pathology

Stories of a Clinical Life

Narrative-Based Practice in Speech-Language Pathology

Stories of a Clinical Life

Jacqueline J. Hinckley, Ph.D., CCC-SLP

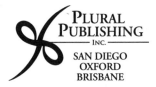

PLURAL
PUBLISHING
INC.

SAN DIEGO
OXFORD
BRISBANE

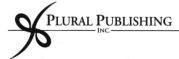
PLURAL PUBLISHING
INC.

5521 Ruffin Road
San Diego, CA 92123

e-mail: info@pluralpublishing.com
Web site: http://www.pluralpublishing.com

49 Bath Street
Abingdon, Oxfordshire OX14 1EA
United Kingdom

Library of Congress Cataloging-in-Publication Data:

Hinckley, Jacqueline J.
    Narrative-based practice in speech-language pathology / Jacqueline Hinckley.
        p. ; cm.
    Includes bibliographical references and index.
    ISBN-13: 978-1-59756-072-6 (pbk.)
    ISBN-10: 1-59756-072-3 (pbk.)
    1. Speech therapy. 2. Narrative medicine. I. Title.
    [DNLM: 1. Language Disorders—therapy. 2. Communication.
3. Professional-Patient Relations. 4. Speech Disorders—therapy. WL 340.2
H659n 2007]
    RC423.H56 2007
    616.85'506—dc22
                                                                2007010305

Contents

Acknowledgments

Like every other clinician, I owe thanks to supervisors and colleagues who shared their experience with me, almost always in the form of stories. There have also been many clients, the names of some are long forgotten, others never forgotten, who have taught me enduring lessons. From among the many people who are characters in my life narrative and made me think in ways that led up to this book, I want to name and thank my husband Ken Schatz, Tom Carr, Carolyn Ellis, Nancy Helm-Estabrooks, Audrey Holland, Colin McPherson, Barb Newborn, Mary Packard, Janet Patterson, Martha Sarno, Annemarie Schuessler, and Herb Silverman.

I also gratefully acknowledge sabbatical support during the academic year 2005–2006, granted by the Provost of the University of South Florida and supported by the Dean and Associate Dean of the College of Arts and Sciences and the Chair of our department. The sabbatical gave me time to think creatively and write productively.

And thanks to Mom, who never tired of reading me the story, "The Little Engine That Could."

Introduction

A twitchy man eyes me and gets in the elevator with me. In the first 2 seconds I am uncomfortable and regret having gotten in the elevator with him. After the doors close and the elevator moves up a couple of floors, he puts a gun to my neck and tells me not to scream.

I think that the man seems nervous enough, maybe crazy enough, to actually shoot me. I realize I might die. "So, Jackie Hinckley is a person who dies at the age of 18," I think to myself. I will never forget the feeling. It was like reading a book without knowing how thick it is or how many more pages are left, and without warning, you discover that you are on the last page of the story. This potential end-of-life realization produced a physical lurch, like taking a step forward when you think the pavement is flat, but abruptly discovering that there's a big step down that you hadn't anticipated.

Thinking that there was nothing else left to lose since I had, at least for the moment, resigned myself to the possibility of immediate death, I began to fight. I pushed him away, and kept pushing and fighting more than he expected. I was able to get past him and scream for help. He immediately ran away.

As it turns out, Jackie Hinckley was not a person who died at the age of 18. She went on to do other things, including writing this book. If you're wondering about the end of this particular story, I wasn't hurt except for a bump on the head. He didn't even take all the money in my purse, so all in all I ended up being a very lucky person who experienced no serious consequences. It was just scary.

The incident, however, lives crystallized in my memory. The first few days after it happened, I retold the sequence of events to police, friends, and neighbors. After that, I ignored it for a while. After a time, I reconsidered what had happened. I started to be able to think how it had affected me and affected the way I think about things. Then I started telling the story again, first to myself, and then to different friends. I no longer simply recounted the events sequentially, like I had to do for the police. I omitted some details, and concentrated the telling of the story to things that were most relevant to its meaningfulness to me. I had decided that it was an event that had forced me to consider the importance of each day, not knowing what might occur on any given day, and that life should be lived knowing that there could be a sudden and unexpected ending. This is not an unusual lesson to learn—everyone does learn it sooner or later. And although such a philosophy is often repeated in various forms, I think most people have an event or series of events in their lives that brings this lesson true meaning and results in a refocusing of their life priorities. I was fortunate to experience such an event at a young age.

So now I have told the story to others many times, and retold it to myself many more times. The circumstances of each retelling have also become a part of the life of the story, and its meaning to me. This is a story that I will remember throughout my life, and if I live to be 80 and tell the story then I will no doubt tell it differently than I did when I was 18. As the years go by, some aspects of the incident are foregrounded, because they contribute more to the meaning I am ascribing to the event, for example, how I felt when the elevator doors closed, or what went through my mind when he pointed the gun at me. Other aspects of the story recede in the telling and also in my memory. For example, I no longer remember what my assailant was wearing, but I do know that I remembered immediately after the event and I was able to tell the police about his clothes. The loss of some of the exact details of the event does not change its meaningfulness to me, nor does it seem to change its meaningfulness to others to whom I tell the story.

This story has become a part of how I think of myself. An important element in the story, when I retell it to myself, is that I was not frozen in fright but chose to fight back. I savor this memory, in an odd way, when times are tough and I want to reassure myself that I can fight my way through adverse circumstances.

The story also contributes to who I think I am as a clinician. I see myself as a "fighter," a person who will struggle through adversity; my clients who see themselves in a similar manner make more natural sense to me than those who are frozen in fear. This is not to say that I don't or can't empathize with clients who have other views. It is simply a reflection of the fact that humans are most congenial when some basic assumptions or perceptions are shared.

I suspect that this story contributes to the way I organize or select therapeutic approaches, too. It is probably no small wonder that my research interest is the development and effectiveness of various therapy approaches; this is probably a reflection of a life theme of mine—to find a way out, to search or fight until circumstances improve.

Each one of my clients has his or her own set of stories that affect, shape, and reflect the story of his or her life. When we come together as clinician and client, our interaction creates its own story. These clinical stories shape and reflect who I am as a clinician, and become a source of learning for myself, my colleagues with whom I share the story, and my students who are just learning about the clinical process.

Speech-language pathologists are uniquely prepared to appreciate and act on a narrative approach to thinking about the identity of our clients and ourselves, and the use of stories to explore the clinical process. We understand the structure of narrative, its development as a linguistic and discourse ability, and the difficulties encountered when clients have impairments that hinder them from normal and complete narrative abilities.

We measure the outcomes of our efforts to intervene in the area of narrative by how well our clients understand and/or produce narratives, and how they use these narrative abilities in various everyday settings such as classrooms and family discussions. But we rarely extend our thinking about narrative to its links with identity. Neither do we often consider its power to reveal the self-defining or at least self-affecting moments that occur during the clinical process.

Narrative can provide a theoretical framework for thinking about identity—the identity of our clients and of ourselves. Narrative is also a tool for exploring our own internal experiences in a way that can be appreciated by others and discussed. Narratives about our experiences as clinicians are likely to contribute to our own definition of ourselves as clinicians. And stories are a powerful tool for persuasion—otherwise and sometimes known as teaching!

The rationale for this book can be summarized in the following three statements.

1. Stories are the way we conceptualize our own identities and the events of our lives and share them with others. We "dream in narrative, daydream in narrative, remember, anticipate, hope, despair, believe, doubt, plan, revise, criticize, construct, gossip, learn, hate and love by narrative" (Hardy, 1986, p. 5). A narrative approach to identity provides a theoretical and conceptual foundation for linking narrative abilities and identity. In short, we live in narrative.

2. Our identity touches the identities of our clients through the clinical process. The clinical process becomes part of our life stories and the life stories of our clients. Thus, moments in the clinical process may be incorporated into our clients' identity and into our own identity as clinicians and as people.

3. Narrative is a framework and a technique with which we can explore the difficult-to-define moments of interaction within the clinical process that have the power to become incorporated into our life stories. These clinical moments hold lessons that we abstract and repeat to ourselves. When shared with colleagues and students, these stories are potential learning moments for others.

The emotional and psychological aspects of the clinical interaction are one of the great remaining frontiers left to explore and study in the discipline of speech-language pathology. This is not to say that no attention has been paid to this component of our daily work. But when we compare ourselves to other related fields, like clinical psychology, occupational therapy, and education, we have paid much less attention to social and emotional processes within the clinical process than our counterparts. It is argued throughout this book that a first step in exploring the great plain of clinical interaction is through understanding, listening to, and telling stories.

Others working in the behavioral sciences also take to telling stories as a way to approach a new or particularly challenging problem.

> The economist Robert Heilbroner once remarked that when forecasts based on economic theory fail, he and his colleagues take to telling stories . . . Narratives may be the last resort of economic theorists. But they are probably the life stuff of those whose behavior they study (Bruner, 1986, pp. 42–43).

Telling stories, it is argued, gets to the "meat" of the matter, particularly when the matter of interest is human behavior, and provides the kernels of truth that frame novel solutions and ideas. How much of our actual accomplishment in sending humans and technology into space or into the depths of the sea is attributable to ideas created and implanted in our mind's eye by science fiction stories? Stories can show things about internal mental life—emotions, plans, reactions—that cannot be adequately interpolated by sheer observation of actions. "Narrative deals with the vicissitudes of human intentions" (Bruner, 1986, p. 16).

Some books are written as a way to show the conclusion of a body of work. Other books are written as a first step in exploring an area, and to hopefully spark interest in a heretofore infrequently discussed area. This book was written with the goal of bringing needed attention to the "clinician side" of the therapeutic equation. In speech-language pathology, we have rightly focused on the client: what client characteristics are associated with particular communication disorders; what the client should do and what kind of service the client needs to achieve particular client goals; what a client's emotional or psychological response might be to a communication disorder, its treatment, and perhaps its chronicity; what counseling techniques are appropriate based on the client's needs; what the client can expect over the long term. There are implications for all of these things for what the clinician should do, of course. Particular suspected diagnoses warrant certain evaluation techniques; specific disorders respond best to certain kinds of treatment offered at particular rates and durations; psychosocial aspects of a client's disorder require the clinician to know when counseling regarding the communication disorder is appropriate and when additional psychological counseling may be best. But we have rarely put our own spotlight on the emotional responses of the clinician, and how these interplay with the client's emotional response or our own selection of treatment procedures. What is the experience of being a clinician? If we assume that the clinical process is an interaction between the client and the clinician, then the question "What is the experience of being a clinician?" is as worthy a question as "What is the experience of having a hearing impairment?" or "What is the experience of being dysfluent?"

The narrative framework provided in this book, and the stories about clinical practice, are offered as one possible route to not only exploring but improving all aspects of our client care.

Plan of the Book

This book is about stories and telling stories. It is about the stories we tell ourselves and tell about ourselves, that define our lives. It is about the stories we tell about ourselves as clinicians, and the stories our clients tell about themselves. It is about how stories about us as clinicians intertwine with and affect the stories our clients tell about themselves.

To talk about stories it is necessary to tell stories. So this book includes stories within the chapters that are examples of important points, and it also includes stories about being a clinician that can stand alone (see Section 3). The stories, by necessity, include me, because my stories are the ones I know best and can tell the best. I don't think that my stories are unique. I think that everyone, and in the case of this book, every clinician, can tell at least as many stories that are important to him or her as I can. Some of your stories might be better or more interesting or more dramatic than my stories. But the point of having my stories in this book is to get you to think about your own stories, and then share them with others, who will very likely in turn share some of their stories with you.

The importance of stories to the development of our life perspective is addressed in Section 1 of the book. Life narrative is important to clinicians and how they perceive their own role as speech-language pathologists. Narrative is also important to how we learn things and how we learn from others. So we will address how clinical stories contribute to professional training and development. Now, each time we work with clients, they also have their own story. They have a story about their life, and a story about their communication disorder. And like the rest of us, they are considering how the story is going to progress in the future. So chapters in the book will also treat how narrative contributes to health and healing, and the development or reconceptualization of the self related to communication disorder.

In Section 2 of the book, the fundamentals of narrative are described so that we can appreciate narrative at a more specific level and also address the kind of conceptual and methodological approach that is being used as a basis for the narratives in this book. Methodologies that are commonly used in a narrative framework are described in Chapter 4, with an emphasis on methods that relate to meta-narratives, life histories, and autoethnography. All of these approaches are rooted in qualitative and ethnographic methods. Illness narratives, or stories about being ill or disabled, have long been studied as a way to describe and understand the experience of ill health. Finally, I review the basics of what we understand about the impact of communication disorders on narrative comprehension and production, and speculate on how we might extend our view of narrative to the formulation of a client's self-view.

Stories that serve as examples of memorable moments in my own clinical development are offered in Section 3. These are provided with discussion questions and background concepts. The intent of these stories is to stimulate discussion. The stories in this section should raise questions and are not intended to provide answers or "morals."

Practical considerations and future directions are considered in Section 4. Areas in which narratives can be used to train clinicians, to enhance professional development, and to facilitate the personal growth of our clients are described. These are offered as a starting point in the hopes that more ideas and practical suggestions will be forthcoming from those of you reading the book and experimenting with the ideas described in it.

Intended Audience

This book is intended for use by clinicians: clinicians-in-training, supervisors, clinical educators, and practicing clinicians at all experience levels. It can be used as a supplementary text in courses on evidence-based practice, professional issues, introduction to clinical practice, or other clinical supervisory courses. It is also designed to be used by the experienced clinician, who is seeking continued professional development and also is required to seek the marker of professional development in the form of Continuing Education Units (CEUs). To facilitate the use of the book in these various learning contexts, each chapter begins with brief summary and specific learning objectives. At the end of each chapter there are study and discussion questions and suggestions for measuring learning outcomes. These can be adapted for classroom use or for use in a professional journal club or independent study by the more experienced clinician. Suggestions and requirements for earning ASHA CEUs through organized journal groups and independent study are summarized in Appendix 1. Always check with ASHA's Web site (http://www.asha.org) for the most current information, policies, and regulations that pertain to earning CEUs.

A Final Word in the Beginning

The stories and anecdotes in this book are mostly my own, and in particular, the stories in Section 3 of the book are my own stories based on my own experiences. I share these with the belief that my experience is typical, not exceptional. I share them because I am hoping that others will be willing to reciprocate and share their stories with me and others around them. I imagine that by sharing our clinical stories the field of speech-language pathology will more formally acknowledge the powerful role of the clinician in the clinical process in professional dialogue and scientific work. The power of the clinician is more than a correctly completed assessment with a matching and well-implemented treatment plan. The power of the clinician is also who you are and who you are to the client. It is time for us to turn our discipline's creative and scientific powers to an important but little-discussed variable in the clinical process—the experience and phenomenon of who you are as a clinician. The conceptual background of a narrative-based approach to clinical practice is offered as one means to accomplish this goal. And, with some trepidation, but knowing that someone must "go first," I offer some of the stories of my clinical life that partially illustrate the potential benefits and rationale of narrative-based practice in speech-language pathology.

Section I

The Importance of Narratives

*"... for no man lives in the external truth,
among salts and acids, but in the warm,
phantasmagoric chamber of his brain, with the
painted windows and the storied walls."*
—Robert L. Stevenson

1

The Development of Identity and Expertise

OVERVIEW

Narrative can be a framework in which we consider our own identities and our identities as clinicians. Our view of ourselves is related to the story we perceive and tell about ourselves. We learn through stories; stories are an important part of how we store and recall knowledge. Stories are argued to be a special case of "instances" for skill acquisition. The story we tell about ourselves as clinicians guides our own clinical comportment.

LEARNING OBJECTIVES

At the end of this chapter, the reader will be able to:

1. Describe procedures for collecting life narratives and self-defining memories.

2. List at least three ways in which stories provide a means for learning.

3. Identify at least one way in which narrative could be used in professional development in speech-language pathology.

Life Narrative

Imagine agreeing to an interview for clinical or research purposes. You sit comfortably in a chair in a pleasant, neutral room. The interviewer smiles and begins.

> I would like you to begin by thinking about your life as if it were a book. Each part of your life composes a chapter in the book. Certainly, the book is unfinished at this point, still, it probably already contains a few interesting and well-defined chapters. Please divide your life into its major chapters and briefly describe each chapter. You may have as many or as few chapters as you like, but I would suggest dividing it into at least two or three chapters and at most about seven or eight. Think of this as a general table of contents for your book. Give each chapter a name and describe the overall contents of each chapter. Discuss briefly what makes for a transition from one chapter to the next. This first part of the interview can expand forever, but I would urge you to keep it relatively brief, say, within thirty to forty-five minutes. Therefore, you don't want to tell me "the whole story" here. Just give me a sense of the story's outline—the major chapters in your life (McAdams, 1993, p. 256).

No doubt, after just a few moments' reflection, you are able to think what those major chapters so far in your life would be. Lifetime periods, such as "my childhood" or "my first marriage," correspond roughly to "main chapters" in a person's life story. Some of my first few chapters would be "growing up," "becoming independent and finding a career," and "working." As I reflect back over my life, I draw the line between chapters at periods that are fairly well demarcated. For example, the transition from "growing up" to "becoming independent and finding a career" was marked by moving away from home. Once I had entered college, also during this chapter, I searched explicitly for a career that I thought I would find rewarding.

According to McAdams' life-story theory of identity, identity is an internalized and evolving life story. Your selection of major chapters in your life reflects your perception of your life story. Because these major chapters reflect such large chunks of life, and because individuals' lives follow similar progressions developmentally and culturally, it is not surprising that many people will identify similar life chapters.

McAdams' interview technique starts with major life chapters as described above and then progresses to an exploration of nuclear episodes. General events like "parties I attended in college" and event-specific knowledge like "the evening I proposed to my wife" have been called nuclear episodes. But these nuclear episodes can also include turning points, high points, and low points.

So, imagine again your comfortable interview room. You have outlined the major chapters of your life story. The interviewer smiles again and continues the interview.

> I am going to ask you about eight key events. A key event should be a specific happening, a critical incident, a significant episode in your past set in a particular time and place. It is helpful to think of such an event as constituting a specific moment in your life that stands out for some reason. Thus, a particular conversation you had with your mother when you were twelve years old or a particular decision you made one afternoon last summer might qualify as a key event in your life story. These are particular moments in a particular time and place, complete with particular characters, actions, thoughts, and feelings. An entire summer vacation—be it very happy or very sad or very important in some way—or a very difficult year in high school, on the other hand, would *not* qualify as key events, because these take place over an extended period

of time. (They are more like life chapters.) For each event, describe in detail what happened, where you were, who was involved, what you did, and what you were thinking and feeling in the event. Also, try to convey the impact this key event has had in your life story and *what this event says about who you are or were as a person*. Did this event change you in any way? If so, in what way? Please be *very specific* here" (McAdams, 1993, p. 258).

The interview goes on to solicit eight key events of the following types: a peak experience, a nadir experience or low point, a turning point, an earliest memory, an important childhood memory, an important adolescent memory, an important adult memory, and one other important memory.

The selection and description of key events or nuclear episodes in your life begins to show in more detail what makes you different from others. A key event in my own life is the time I was robbed at gunpoint, as described in the Introduction. The memory of this event, and its retelling both to me and to others, has changed over the years, and probably will continue to change. The selection of key events is a way of making sense out of things that have happened to you. You select the events that seem most meaningful to you, and you chain them together in a personally meaningful way. Similarly, you will select details and descriptions of the event in a way that renders it important to your own identity. As McAdams writes,

> To a certain degree, then, identity is a product of choice. We choose the events that we consider most important for defining who we are and providing our lives with some semblance of unity and purpose, and we endow them with symbolism, lessons learned, integrative themes, and other personal meanings that make sense to us in the present as we survey the past and anticipate the future (McAdams, 2003, p. 196).

Imagine your interviewer next asks you about *significant people*, that is, the cast of characters in your life. Once you have established the main chapters and the key events, it is appropriate to describe in more detail the family members, spouse, friends, mentors, teachers, or others who have had a profound impact on who you think you are as a person. In the structured interview technique, you are asked to describe at least four significant people in your life, at least one of whom should not be a relative (McAdams, 1993).

The fourth and final segment of the interview is to ask you about your future plans and goals. What hopes, dreams, and aspirations do you have? How does the story that you have written so far continue into the future? How do you currently envision the future chapters of the story?

Alternatives to the life-story theory of identity include Freud's contention that personality development occurs in the early childhood years, and Erikson's views of stages of development during which identity is a primary issue during adolescence and early adulthood. There are many other psychological theories on identity, and arguments and evidence for and against various views. It is not the purpose of this book to review all of these theories, nor to detail any particular account of identity or identity formation. Rather, the primary purpose of this book is to show how stories and their telling intersect with our own identities as a person, and with our identities as clinicians. Each of us can tell a story not only of our whole life, but a story of ourselves as developing clinicians. We might divide such a story of ourselves as clinicians into chapters, beginning with "training" to "current job with 20 years of experience." Key events—high points, low points, turning points—of our working lives as clinicians can be recalled and specifically described and are often retold to ourselves and to others. There are significant people in the story of our lives as clinicians—teachers, supervisors, colleagues. And finally we have future goals, plans, and hopes for who we would like to be as clinicians. All of this, of course, is part of who we think we are as people.

Our clients, too, whether young children or older adults, male or female, with multiple disabilities or with a single, specific communication disorder, have their own stories to tell about their lives. Some of these clients will identify chapters in their lives relevant to their communication disorder—for example, "my stroke and aphasia." Others among our clients will have integrated the communication disorder into their view of themselves so that the communication disorder is not a chapter, but it is a theme that runs throughout the major chapters and key events of their lives. The significant cast of characters in our clients' stories may change after the sudden onset of a communication disorder, or their roles may change. When a communication disorder is present early in life, some significant people may remain the same but may need to change their roles in relation to the developmental process.

For a couple of hours a week for a few weeks or so, who I am as a person and as a clinician intersects with who my client is as a person and who they think they should be as a client. This intertwining of our stories creates its own story. Some of these intersections become key events in the story of myself as a person and as a clinician. And perhaps, some of these hours also become key events in the stories of the lives of my clients.

This book is about stories—the stories we tell about ourselves as people, the stories we tell about ourselves in particular roles as clinicians and clients, and the stories of the intricate dance between the two as we come together in the clinical process.

Using Stories to Create Identity

According to some theorists and researchers, telling the story of one's life, as you might do in an interview, is a process that has developed over the course of the life span. These theorists, McAdams for example, argue that we learn to think of our own identity through a narrative process (Bateson, 1989; Cohler, 1982; Eakin, 1999; McAdams, 1996; Neiser, 1993; Neiser & Jopling, 1997; Olney, 1998; Schriffin, 1996).

As speech-language pathologists, we are well aware of the nature and importance of narrative and narrative discourse to the functional communication abilities of our clients. We do not often extend knowledge of narrative and narrative abilities to thinking about the development or reformulation of our client's identity. Nor do we typically apply our understanding of narrative to thinking about our own role as therapists in the clinical process.

The narrative approach to creating one's identity may well begin in the earliest childhood days, even before children can follow the most basic story (McAdams, 1993). Most developmental psychologists agree that during the first year or two of life, early relationships between the child and the caregivers help to develop general attitudes and views of the world, especially of others in the world. Are others trustworthy or consistent? Are there attention, nurturing, and affection in the world? These fundamental perceptions developed early in life contribute to what McAdams calls *narrative tone*. Is the story of your life an optimistic or hopeful one? Then perhaps those early years contributed to a positive narrative tone.

It is easier to observe the relationship between stories and the development of the self after the ages of 3, 4, or 5 years, as children begin listening and responding to stories, and ultimately choosing particular stories and then producing their own. Children hear stories, most often in the form of fables and fairy tales. As children become able to listen to and understand stories, they start to select the reading of particular stories. Sometimes children want to hear the same story over and over again.

According to Bettelheim, children request repeated readings of stories when that particular story is especially meaningful in some way to an issue that the child is working out at that time (Bettelheim, 1976). Children develop favorite stories or favorite parts of particular stories, and this may reflect aspects of their cognitive development and development of their own identity.

Children listen to stories and identify the good and the bad characters in the story and the good and bad events and actions. It has been suggested that children listen to stories and think about whether they would like to be good or bad. Once that question is answered, the child then comes to the conclusion that to be good, one should be like the good character. They pose the question, "What do I want to be like?" and then answer it with, "So I'll be like this or that character." A favorite story of my own mother's was "The Little Engine That Could," and I loved it, too. I heard that story and read it myself probably hundreds of times as a child. It would not be at all surprising to find that many clinicians and others who work with those with special needs found particular meaning in that story or another one with a similar theme. Being judged as too small or not strong enough or in some other way not right to accomplish the goal, but then being able to slowly, painstakingly make the top of the mountain is a theme that reflects the heart of our profession and is likely to be a preferred theme for many of us.

As we develop through childhood and adolescence, we excel in our ability to tell our own stories. First we tell the simple story that recounts the particulars of a special event, day at school, or family outing. Our stories become more complex, and by adolescence we can spend hours and hours on the phone each day telling stories about who said what to whom and what would happen if he liked her. This period is a transition from what has been called the *prenarrative era* of one's life to the *narrative era*. During adolescence and into the young adult years, the explicit question, "Who am I?" is typically articulated and explored. Very often potential future chapters of one's story are tried on for size during this period. Do I want to grow up and get a job? Raise a family? Become a world traveler? Tour the country as a rodeo clown? As Jerome Bruner wrote, "Self-making is a narrative art" (Bruner, 2003, p. 210). Stories are convenient means by which we can try on alternative endings.

The story that develops is one that encompasses previous life chapters and key events, and also has tentative plans for the kinds of chapters that will become part of the story in the future. The story that develops must be one in which the protagonist is oneself, acting in the real, grown-up world. McAdams (1993) defines identity as an integrative configuration of self-in-the-adult-world. When we hit upon a story of ourselves acting in the world in a way that makes sense and is pleasing to us, identity has been shaped. Recently I saw a bumper sticker that read "My life is based on a true story." Although there may be many levels of meanings to that slogan, one interpretation is consistent with the life narrative approach to identity.

We develop an idealized personification of the self, and this image (or *imago*, according to McAdams, 1984) becomes the main characters in our own developing life narrative. "One's life becomes a story with a large cast of self-characters who assume different positions in the narrative, take on different voices, represent different self-facets, personify significant trends during different developmental chapters—all in the same evolving story, the same identity" (Hermans, 1996, p. 226).

As time passes, events occur, and life develops, the story changes to meet the needs of the aging protagonist. "Consequently, it should not be surprising to observe considerable revising and reworking of one's life story, even the reimagining of the distant past, in light of changing psychosocial concerns in the adult years and changing understandings of what the near and distant future may bring" (McAdams, 2003, p. 194). This "reworking" of the life story can become a problem-solving technique, in the sense that different future chapters or story lines can be imagined and "tried on for size." In the story I related in the Introduction to this book, the traumatic event of being at gunpoint forced me to quickly consider an alternate end to my own life story that I had not previously considered. But under less traumatic circumstances, we can imagine ourselves in different places, doing different jobs, living in a different way, and visualize how such a story would work for our protagonist—ourselves. According to Paul Ricoeur (Ricoeur, 1983), stories are "models for the redescription of the world."

As experience gathers, some memories become self-defining memories. Some event, and the story that we have shaped around the event, becomes something that we retell to ourselves and perhaps to others. Our own actions, the character and role we played out in the story, becomes a memory on which we may base future decisions or actions (Pillemer, 1998; Woike, 1995). Nelson (1993) describes these memories this way: "Self-defining memories, like all personal memories, concern specific and memorable past events." Self-defining memories are further described as "particularly vivid, emotional, and familiar, revealing 'affective patterns and themes that stamp an individual's most important concerns'" (Singer & Salovey, 1993, p. 4).

Not only are self-defining memories critical to one's own development of identity, but they become "nuggets" or shorthand methods for sharing with others critical characteristics of ourselves (Thorne & McLean, 2003). An anecdote about something that has happened and how we acted under that particular set of circumstances can tell another person a lot about how we might be expected to respond in certain situations. But perhaps most of all, a story we tell about ourselves is a story that we have created and edited, and it tells other people what we would like to think about ourselves, or perhaps what we would like others to think of us.

Life narrative theorists and investigators use various techniques for collecting not just overall life stories, but also for collecting self-defining memories. Typically, a participant would be asked to relate a memory that meets the following description.

1. It is a personal memory that is *at least 1 year old*.
2. It is highly *vivid*.
3. The memory continues to *evoke strong feelings* even now.
4. The memory "convey(s) powerfully *how you have come to be the person you currently are*" (Singer & Moffitt, 1991–1992, p. 242, emphasis added).

The 1-year-old age requirement for the memory to be told as a self-defining memory is based on the idea that, for a memory to affect one's identity or to become incorporated into one's own identity, time must pass. The memory must be "digested," allowed to roll around in the head and bounce up against other previous memories and ideas about one's own identity (Ricoeur, 1991).

A self-defining memory must be *vivid*, *evocative*, and judged as demonstrating *important self characteristics* by the teller. If it is vivid in one's own memory, this lends credence to its importance and to how much the teller may have rehearsed this memory to him- or herself. Evocative memories are those that are likely to create similar emotions in a hearer of the story, and thus such a memory or story serves the purpose of sharing with another person the way you felt under a specific set of circumstances. Both of these are intertwined, of course, with one's own judgment that the memory and its story illustrate some aspect of how one thinks of oneself.

When researchers in the area of life narratives and self-defining memories collect stories from participants, they may differentiate the event narrative from the telling narrative. The event narrative is retelling the sequence of events that constitute a self-defining memory. The telling narrative is how, when, and why the event was told to someone else. The telling narrative is more likely to include the evaluative component of the event—why the event is self-defining, why it has remained important to the individual's identity. So, in addition to asking a participant to share a self-defining memory that meets the four characteristics above, the participant is also asked to tell about a time when he shared that story with someone else. To whom did you tell it? Under what set of circumstances? Why did you tell this person? What happened?

Social and Cultural Roots of Life Stories

Life stories are told to others—family, friends; they are socially constructed (Pasaputhi, 2006). This aspect of life stories is inherent in the definition of self-defining memories and the techniques used to solicit them. The first time you retell a sequence of events to a friend, your friend may ask you questions or react in ways that you may or may not have expected. This might lead you to consider the event in a slightly different way, and the event may change in its meaning for you as a result of this social interaction. The second time you tell this story to a different person, you may revise your telling of it, in either subtle ways or major ways, to accommodate the new meaning created from the first time you told the story. As Carbaugh (1996, pp. 213–214) wrote: "Identities are something created and subjected to particular conversational dynamics. . . . From this vantage point the question 'Who am I?' depends partly on 'where I am,' 'with whom I am,' and material and symbolic resources that are available to the people there."

This social construction is a joint, interactive process; it is not one in which another interprets for you or tells you the meaning of your story. Bettelheim argues that the child must contemplate the problem in any story and the possible solutions independently, in order to feel a sense of achievement and mastery. He concludes his argument: "We grow, we find meaning in life, and security in ourselves by having understood and solved personal problems on our own, not by having them explained to us by others" (Bettelheim, 1976, pp. 18–19).

Indeed, it has been argued by many that understanding narrative and being able to participate in narrative allow us to interact socially with those around us. Imagining and processing stories allows us to have a sense of self and a sense of others. Culture provides a set of expectations for what others are likely to act or feel and this creates the scenery against which we create our life narrative. Bruner concludes, as he argues this point, that "Again, life could be said to imitate art" (Bruner, 1986, p. 69).

The cultural context not only provides a set of expectations for how others around us might act or react, but also provides a set of expectations regarding how a story is told. The cultural context will provide a sense of when it is appropriate to tell the story and to whom the story can or should be told. We will tell the story with a structure, style, and technique that is consistent with our culture. In fact, one definition of community is a group of people with a shared narrative. Much has been written about the narrative forms used in various cultures, and the intent is not to review that literature here. (See Appendix 2 for a list of key reviews and references in this area.) Rather, we recognize that social construction of stories and the cultural context in which the story lives plays a role in how stories shape our own identities.

So our stories, while conforming to cultural and social expectations, can be thought of as efforts to distinguish ourselves, to show our own individuality. As stated by Thorne and MacLean,

" 'Culture' presses us to consider how people are similar, whereas 'self' presses us to consider the uniqueness of individual lives" (Thorne & McLean, 2003, p. 169).

An interesting counterexample illustrates how expectations from the social and cultural context can be differentiated from the development of our own individual identities (Byrne, 2003). Byrne describes the case of a young woman in psychotherapy who was asked to tell the story of her life. She began by indicating that she had no story to tell. Her mother, however, was quite happy to provide the story of her daughter's life. The therapist came to the conclusion that the young woman was acting out a role in a story narrated by her mother, rather than creating her own life story. If an individual seems not to have a story to tell, it is perhaps because the person is so concerned that his or her life conforms to expected and perceived social and cultural norms there seems not to be any press to differentiate oneself from the canonical sociocultural expectations.

Learning Through Listening to Stories

Children identify with characters in stories and thus learn about characters' qualities and choices, and from there may develop their own sense of identity. As children grow into adults, there is no reason to think that this ability to project oneself into a story and learn from it is lost. On the contrary, much has been written about case-based learning and learning through anecdotes. Entire university curricula are now being designed around cases, case study, and the in-depth exploration of the ramifications of individual cases.

We learn from stories, case stories, and anecdotes, by considering the details available in a scenario and drawing broad conclusions from it. In contrast to learning general rules or guidelines, learning from cases or stories allows us to consider explicitly the role of particular variables and details and how these variables interact with the general principles we are learning or trying to abstract from the case. How is a communication diagnosis affected by a negative developmental or medical history, versus the ramifications of a complex medical history with multiple injuries or diseases? How is an intervention plan specifically affected when the client is a school-age child versus a retired adult? In addition to the consideration of case details, the learner imagines him- or herself in the position of protagonist. What would she do in that set of circumstances? How would he feel if a client responded in the way it happened in the story being told?

Stories are a powerful means to try out alternatives both for the development of the child and the continued learning of the adult. Bruner (1986) describes the role of stories in development and learning in this way:

> For stories define the range of canonical characters, the settings in which they operate, the actions that are permissible and comprehensible. And thereby they provide, so to speak, a map of possible roles and of possible worlds in which action, thought and self-definition are permissible (or desirable). As we enter more actively into the life of a culture around us, as Victor Turner remarks, we come increasingly to play parts defined by the "dramas" of that culture. Indeed, in time the young entrant into the culture comes to define his own intentions and even his own history in terms of the characteristic cultural dramas in which he plays a part—at first family dramas, but later the ones that share the expanding circle of his activities outside the family (pp. 66–67).

The drama of stories stays with us. Stories are whole "memory chunks" that can be indelibly inked on our brains. As a middle-aged woman, I still remember the story my mother told me when I was a small child in the bathtub. She told me about a little girl who never remembered to wash her neck. Her neck became black with dirt even though the rest of her was clean. All the other children at school started to tease her because she had such a dirty neck. This story still crosses my mind sometimes, while washing my neck. The message my mother wanted to get across to me was more powerfully communicated because I could imagine this little girl who was being teased at school for lack of good scrubbing. I did not want to be a girl like that! My mother barely if at all remembers telling me this story; but as a young listener I was strongly affected.

As adults we continue to seek out examples of others who have already done things we are considering, and we look to those with more experience to tell us stories from which we might gain insight about things we have not yet tried. Stories of actual experiences are often taken more seriously than general pronouncements.

Stories provide details that we can match to our own set of circumstances, allowing us to weigh how much a particular person's experience might map onto our own. Rules, guidelines, or general conclusions cannot accommodate special characteristics of individual exemplars.

Stories also allow one to consider alternative "possible worlds" (Bruner, 1986). We can investigate, speculate, and consider alternative routes to a desired ending. Hearing multiple stories about a similar subject enables us to differentiate details that led to various endings.

> As every narrative, self-account is itself part of a life, embedded in a lived context of interaction and communication, intention and imagination, ambiguity and vagueness, there is always potentially, a next and different story to tell, as there occur different situations in which to tell it. This creates a dynamic that keeps in view actual stories about real life with possible stories about potential life, as well as combinations of them. As a consequence, life narratives, like most literary texts, can be treated as open, without end. They are, as Bakhtin (1981) puts it, "unfinalizable," for life always opens up more options ("real" and "fictional" ones), includes more meanings, more identities, evokes more interpretations than even the number of all possible life stories could express. . . . Viewed in this way, we may conclude that the study of life narratives is not only wedded to actual and particular human life worlds, but turns into a laboratory of possibilities for human identity construction (Brockmeier & Carbaugh, 2001, pp. 7–8).

Multiple stories also allow us to abstract similarities, to store cues and responses against the backdrop of a detailed context. Which actions seem to consistently produce certain outcomes, in spite of variations in the context? Are there actions that seem important but seem not to be related to a desired outcome? As a sailor, I have heard many stories about people sailing into all kinds of situations, on a particular type of boat, and from their experience the storyteller insists that their route is the only way to get there from here, or this piece of equipment is the only way to accomplish a certain goal, or one should always go by this or that weather report. After hearing at least hundreds of these stories, many of which have been about similar places or similar conditions, I can only come to the conclusion that everyone seems to take slightly different actions and use different equipment and all of these variations produce the same outcome—people arrive in the place they wanted to go to, for the most part. In this case, the variety of details precludes any generalizations, except to say that everyone, in different boats and in different ways, sails on.

Learning Through Anecdotes

Psychological theories provide a foundation for a deeper understanding of how we learn through anecdotes, stories, and examples. The role of stories as a type of knowledge structure and a means by which we store and retrieve information in memory has been thoroughly argued (e.g., Conway & Pleydell-Pearce, 2000; Neiser & Fivush, 1996). According to Schank and Abelson (1977; 1995; and Schank, 1991), virtually all of what we know is stored in the form of stories. When we encounter new information—also in the form of stories—the new stories are integrated into already existing stories. Finally, stories are socially constructed through retelling, and the retelling of stories contributes to our sense of self.

Another important contributor to the development of theories having to do with this kind of learning, or instance-based learning, is Gordon Logan (Logan, 1988; 2002). Instance-based learning is a developed theory that posits that the experience of each "instance," or example of an event, contributes to the development of general responses to a set of contextual cues.

An instance is an event that is characterized by all of its contextual cues—sensory cues and sociocultural cues. As we encounter the next instance, cues and conditions that are similar to the first instance are strengthened. Thus similar, repeated cues and conditions become strongly associated with actions and responses within the instance.

Instance-based theories of skill acquisition are differentiated from componential learning approaches in which small portions of a more complex skill or context are broken down and trained separately. In instance-based theories, the richness of the context is critical for laying down important memories and being able to later retrieve learned strategies or information based on cues that may be variable across contexts.

Specific training examples that parallel instance-based theory come from the whole-task training literature. In whole-task training, an entire context including procedures in their typical sequence, and thus typical cues and corresponding actions and reactions, are trained repeatedly. This is contrasted with part-task training, in which the component parts of a skill or procedure are practiced separately, and then later combined together in the complete context.

Both part-task and whole-task training are used when training pilots or others who must attend to multiple complex items quickly. Training may occur on a single instrument or small group of instruments, but whole-task training must also occur in which the pilot trainee practices attending to and analyzing data from all of the typical instruments available on the flight deck, and making appropriate responses. Thus, the government has invested in research comparing part-task and whole-task training for a variety of complex tasks that need to be accomplished by those in military service.

Part-task and whole-task training have also been compared for children and adults with various disabilities. A vocational task, threading an industrial sewing machine, was used as a training context with adults with developmental disabilities (Nettlebeck & Kirby, 1976). Adults were either trained in part-task or whole-task training. The part-task training broke down the threading to individual steps, and each step of threading the sewing machine was trained separately. They were combined later only after criterion was reached for each individual step. The whole-task training involved going through all of the steps of the training in sequence at each training encounter. Those adults with disabilities who participated in the whole-task training required more trials initially to demonstrate mastery, but ultimately demonstrated the ability to thread the sewing machine in overall fewer learning trials, and the learning appeared to be more robust over time compared to those who underwent the part-task training.

A story, it could be argued, is an instance. A story has all of the contextual details, explicitly stated, implied, or imagined, that a real event does, without certain sensorial experiences. A story depicts intentions, actions, and emotional reactions in such a way that these are linked to the contextual cues within the story. Hearing a story, particularly when it is about a particular experience relevant to our own, carries at least some of the weight of an actually experienced instance.

It is not far-fetched to argue that hearing stories that result in imagining ourselves in the protagonist's position produces similar results to being in the actual experience. Visualization and imagery have long been used by premier athletes as training tools to achieve success. In multiple contexts, visualizing an action, for example moving an arm, has been shown to produce activation in some of the same brain regions as the actual movement does. Listening to verbal descriptions produces some overlap in brain region activation as recalling images formed based on previously experienced perception (for a review, see Cocude, Mellet, & Denis, 1999). So, when we imagine ourselves performing actions, it is possible that we are producing similar physiological patterns as when we actually do those actions.

Stories provide a means to imagine ourselves in a variety of circumstances and learn from those circumstances and the outcomes without actually having to experience every possibility. We store information about the contextual cues linked to the various actions, and when we come upon those cues again, either in a story or in real life, the cues should trigger a link to responses. The more stories we hear, the more generalizations we build. The more stories we hear, the more flexibility of response we develop, because we acquire sensitivity to a variety of cues and develop a repertoire of actions linked to these cues.

Learning from stories may appear slower at the outset, because the basic foundation, which is a component part of the knowledge base that is being built, has not yet been laid, and this foundation must be built by the learner across a variety of cases or stories. But the learning that comes from stories is more flexible and more robust over time. Thus stories are the near-equivalent of experience as a learning mechanism.

Telling our own stories is also a form of learning. As children we learned the canonical forms for storytelling and the appropriate social and cultural contexts. We learn to tell stories in a way that matches the expectations of those around us, and yet we present ourselves through our stories in a way that is pleasing to us, and in the way that we would like others to perceive us. We learn about ourselves through the telling of particular incidents and the social creation of the story, which varies somewhat each time we tell it. Sometimes, it is only after we have found ourselves telling the story of a particular event more than once that we realize the significance of that incident to ourselves. The story becomes meaningful, and we learn from it, through the telling of it.

A Clinical Life Narrative

Just as we develop our own identity as a person through narrative, we develop our own identity as a clinician through narrative, too. We hear stories that others share with us, we hear stories about other clinicians, and we formulate our own stories about our lives as a clinician. Through these stories we develop a clinical identity, an image of ourselves as a clinician. We become the protagonist who is a speech-language pathologist in the daily story of working as a clinician.

Now you may be thinking to yourself that a narrative approach to identity development—our identity either as a whole person or our identity as a clinician—makes very nice sense but seems awfully "subjective." Is there really a place for this kind of discussion in the discipline of speech-language pathology? Those of us who are trained in the scientific method have been taught to be distrustful of self-reported data and, in particular, self-reported data from long in the past. Most of us, as speech-language pathologists, are dutifully entrenched in the idea that data must be "fresh," immediate; evaluations should be repeated if too far in the past so that a more realistic current picture of abilities is available to us; references cited should be recent; and subjective memory, without corroborating evidence, is not to be trusted. These are all good and important principles and hold an important place in the practice of our profession. But our ability to embrace these concepts should not lead to our complete exclusion of things that do not comply with these guidelines, particularly when purposes differ.

Applying the scientific method and scientific principles are critical to supporting proposed hypotheses or verifying theories. Matching diagnoses and severity levels with appropriate interventions, for example, certainly should be an evidence-based process, based on data collected according to the scientific method. Not all of our clinical work, however, is subject to hypotheses and theories. How to best greet our client who we suspect is showing signs of depression, or how to artfully inform parents about the kinds of services that will be best for their child who they desperately hope does not have a disability of any kind, are aspects of our clinical work for which no amount of hypotheses, theories, or scientific method-based work will suffice. To learn to be a good clinician in difficult clinical interactions of these kinds, we must use what we know about being human from our own experience, what we have heard about from others' experience, and what we have observed during training and professional development opportunities.

Stories are a powerful means of developing the art of clinical interaction. We can become more skilled at various aspects of clinical work by telling and listening to stories. The set of characteristics that we believe defines us as people and specifically in our role as a clinician will guide our reactions to our clients. We set up a set of expectations without ourselves for how we believe a "good" clinician should react, and as we develop experience, a set of expectations for how we believe we typically react to a certain set of clinical circumstances. Do we see ourselves as an authority figure, whose primary role is to impart information? Is our clinical identity tied to being a sympathetic helper? A special kind of teacher? Our self-perceptions will color our responses to our clients. Sometimes, our perceptions of our role as a clinician match our client's perception of our role as a clinician, and other times, there is a mismatch. In any case, awareness of our perceived identity as a clinician can make us more alert to how our actions fit with our clients' expectations, and may improve our flexibility in adapting to the differing roles that serve various clients optimally.

Evidence-based practice is crucial, but it results in broad-based generalizations and overall conclusions. These are critical to the development of practice guidelines and standards. But stories balance the scales, and help convey the information about individuality that is purposefully "washed out" in large-scale studies. A narrative approach on the one hand, and evidence-based practice on the other, provides a balance between the art and the science of clinical practice.

Listening to Others' Clinical Stories

As the child first listens to fables and fairy tales, the adult who is beginning his or her clinical career also wants to listen to stories. Clinical stories help to paint the landscape of clinical work, and enable the student to imagine him- or herself in the role of clinician, trying it on for size. The question, "What is it like to be a speech-language pathologist?" is probably most effectively answered with a few well-chosen stories of clinical work. As stated by Brockmeir and Harre: "Narrative, we suspect, is the most powerful mode of persuasion" (Brockmeir & Harre, 2001, p. 41). Responses to such a question that are more general, such as "It is very rewarding," are fine but probably not what the person who posed that question is really looking for as a response.

As clinicians develop, they can start to compare their own experiences with others' clinical stories. More knowledge and experience will enable the clinician to interact with others' stories more actively, as they imagine themselves in the protagonist's role. The more experienced a clinician becomes, the more others' stories can be an opportunity to project oneself in a set of circumstances, some of which may already be familiar. In this case, the contextual cues of a heard story may trigger a link to an already established action or response. If the recalled action or response to that kind of circumstance is different from the story as it progresses, this is an opportunity for the experienced clinician to draw fine points of distinction or enhance one's own repertoire of clinical responses.

The tradition of "case studies" or "clinical anecdotes" is well established in the history of the practice of medicine, and in the last century this tradition has been extended to allied health including speech-language pathology. It has long been common practice in medical schools and teaching hospitals to hold "grand rounds," in which a case example is reviewed in detail including medical diagnoses, procedures, and treatments. In all of these cases, the story of that individual case is narrated by the presenting student or physician, and it is anticipated that those in attendance will learn from listening to this particular story.

More recently, the advantages of case-based learning have been explored in the pedagogical literature. Whole university curricula for some disciplines, including speech-language pathology and related fields like physical therapy, have been designed to be completely based on learning groups that deeply investigate a well-chosen series of cases that are exemplars of various clinical characteristics or techniques. Instead of taking an introductory course on phonology, for example, students in such a curriculum encounter a case of phonological disorder and, usually in learning teams with a mentor, study the principles and strategies necessary to understand the nature of the disorder and its treatment.

The advantages of such a curriculum are usually described in terms of problem-solving ability, reflecting the flexibility of knowledge that develops from exposure to rich contexts in addition to the experiential aspect of our clinical training. It may be that this problem-solving ability extends to clinical interactions and the handling of challenging clinical situations. The student who is exposed to in-depth case study, in addition to typical amounts of clinical practica assignments, may store and be able to retrieve a variety of actions including interpersonal skills in response to contextual cues that are superior, over the course of the training period, than those students whose coursework is presented in a more traditional format and who must rely solely on practica experiences for the learning of clinical interaction skills.

As more experienced clinicians, we may also be able to judge the development of our clinicians-in-training in a richer way by asking them to tell us their own clinical stories, requiring them to reflect on their experiences and measure their performance against the social and cultural expectations of our discipline which they are also developing. Students who can give multiple examples or stories to illustrate a particular lesson learned, procedure, or technique may have mastered that knowledge more fully than the student who can generate only a single exemplar.

The more experienced we become, the more our stories become meaningful to us as we reflect back and retell the stories. These *self-defining* stories—stories that are particularly important to us as we look back on our developing clinical identities—are likely to be important in some way to others who listen to them. These stories are rich in detail, have been created socially through multiple retellings, and have the benefit of our retrospective view of what they have taught us. When others—regardless of experience level—listen to these stories, they learn from our experience by absorbing the contextual detail and the story of our actions. Even without a specific interpretation, such a story can leave a powerful impression.

Telling Stories about Oneself as a Clinician

All of us who are speech-language pathologists share certain elements of the story we tell about ourselves and in particular the story of ourselves as clinicians. First, we are likely to share elements of the stories about our identities because we have chosen a helping profession, and this kind of chapter in a life story makes sense when it derives from certain kinds of preceding chapters. Second, we have all shared very similar training as we began in this field, and this is especially true in countries where national certifying or licensing agencies set training standards.

Adults who are distinguished as parents, teachers, volunteers, and other helpers and community leaders have been observed to share major themes in their life stories—described as a "commitment story" by McAdams (McAdams, Diamond, de St. Aubin, & Manfield, 1997). This commitment story is characterized by certain common elements. First, the protagonist may enjoy an early family advantage, or at least perceives an advantage of some kind. Next, the protagonist becomes sensitized to the suffering of others at an early age, perhaps through events within his or her own family, extended family, or other compelling experience. The helping adult who tells a commitment story tends to be guided by clear and compelling personal ideology that remains relatively stable over time. The commitment story continues with a "redemption sequence"—the transformation of bad scenes into good outcomes. The final element of the commitment story is that the protagonist sets goals for the future that will benefit society. It would be interesting to know how many of us in speech-language pathology would spontaneously share a life narrative that contains these basic elements of the commitment story.

Our common training backgrounds tend to ensure that aspects of our stories as clinicians are shared. We learn what is expected in the culture of speech-language pathology. These cultural expectations might vary somewhat depending on our ultimate particular work circumstances (e.g., schools, hospitals, etc.) but in general we share a set of expectations that guide the way we do our clinical work. We share a set of ethical standards, common knowledge about the goals and domains of our discipline, and an understanding of how speech-language pathologists are expected to act and portray themselves professionally.

Against the backdrop of our professional culture, we strive ultimately to distinguish ourselves as individuals, to find our own identities as clinicians. Stories about our personal experiences, our self-defining moments as clinicians, or stories that illustrate typical situations, serve to describe ourselves as clinicians both to ourselves and to others. We generate stories about ourselves as clinicians and enjoy the telling of them to colleagues who can appreciate and share our professional culture and knowledge base. As we tell these stories, we create a sense of identity as clinicians. It is this identity that guides us in our clinical interactions and intertwines with our clients' identity. Ultimately, new meaningful moments—self-defining stories and memories—are created that impact our own identity and that of our clients.

STUDY/DISCUSSION QUESTIONS AND ACTIVITIES

1. Provide one personal example of a self-defining memory. Make sure that it meets the criteria described in the chapter.
2. How does this story of a self-defining memory reflect your social and cultural background and expectations?
3. In what ways does this self-defining memory identify you as an individual? What does it say about you?
4. Is there a client who frequently selected or retold the same story repeatedly? How was this story meaningful to that client? Was this story a reflection of the client as an individual in some way?

2

Health, Healing, and Stories

OVERVIEW

This chapter summarizes the links between narrative and healing and health. Individuals who tell stories about stressful life events generally maintain better health. Individuals who are ill also gain positive benefits from narrative. Benefits from telling stories about anxiety-producing events include improvements in physical health and psychological health. Perhaps the most robust outcome related to telling stories about emotional events is an improvement in coping mechanisms. Narratives enable the individual to create meaning and coherence during times of disruption, chaos, and unpredictability.

LEARNING OBJECTIVES

At the end of this chapter, the reader will be able to:

1. Describe the conceptual origins of a narrative-based approach.

2. Define *deconstruction* as it is applied to narrative therapy.

3. List the critical features of a therapeutic expressive writing paradigm.

4. Identify at least three physical or psychological health outcomes that have been linked to narrative-based interventions.

Positive Health Benefits of Narrative

As events unfold in our lives, we weave a story in which we are the protagonist, thus creating connections between past and current life events and future hopes and plans. Each individual's story, as created by the narrator, will reveal an overall tone and also tend to point towards a certain kind of denouement—a happy or sad ending. Stories can provide hope—they can help one conceptualize potential alternative solutions or endings to a problem.

The potential for stories to save us from others' actions or our own actions has been a theme through the ages. The motif in "Thousand and One Nights" is the power of stories to save; the virgin saves herself and others by telling a story that continues for a thousand nights. In other substories other characters save themselves through the telling of stories. We often preserve our own ego, maintain optimism, inspire hope, and encourage others through stories.

This potential for hope and the possibility of narrating one's own story in a positive manner have effects on our emotional, psychological, and physical health. The field of psychoneuroimmunology has shown the seamlessness between our psychological selves and our physical selves. We know that social support and positive attitude produce measurable effects on our general health as well as recovery from illness. So stories, inasmuch as they are a way to meaningfulness and to framing a potential positive future, play a role in how we accommodate life events, in either a healthy or unhealthy way. And stories also contribute to adjustment to injury or illness or disability and thus long-term health after the onset of these physical changes.

Recently, the National Endowment for the Arts has funded Operation: Homecoming, a project that provides workshops and encouragement for soldiers to write about their current war experiences. John Peede, director of the project, says high-ranking officers are often very supportive of such writing projects. "Because they know it's healthy to tell these stories. Notice I say: it's healthy. It's not easy" (*Miami Herald*, November 14, 2005). Even national funding organizations and representatives of the military services are acknowledging that there are positive health benefits from telling one's own story. From this project, stories about war experiences have emerged on blogs, and a few book projects have developed, full of the stories of how these young men adapt to traumatic experiences.

Stories of life events, mundane or traumatic events, can be told in various ways. Individuals can turn bad events into positive outcomes in a story, or can tell what might otherwise be considered a good event in a way that has a bad ending. McAdams (McAdams, de St. Aubin, & Logan, 1993; McAdams, 1999) contrasts redemption sequences in life stories (bad scenes transformed into good outcomes) with contamination sequences (an emotionally positive event goes suddenly bad). Redemption sequences in life stories are positively associated with self-reported measures of life satisfaction, self-esteem, and sense of life coherence, and negatively associated with depression. Contamination sequences are positively associated with depression and negatively associated with life satisfaction, self-esteem, and sense of life coherence. This observation is consistent with the literature in health psychology showing that people who report benefits following their injuries, illnesses, or misfortunes tend to show faster recovery from their setbacks and more positive well-being overall (Affleck & Tennen, 1996). Life-story telling functions to provide the self with identity and also can be instrumental in the overall maintenance of mental health.

The power of stories for healing from illness has a long history as well as current application. In Hindu medicine, the mentally deranged person is told a fairy tale, contemplation of which will help him overcome his emotional disturbance. This is a clear example of the use of a positive story, or adapting and creating a favorable version of a series of life events, to promote well-being. Most folks adapt to life events by creating their own positive story. But in the case of those who cannot or do not generate a positive life story, well-being may be facilitated by offering a positive story that fits that individual's life circumstances.

Creating a narrative out of life events not only provides the opportunity to attach events to an overall positive tone, but also may provide some sense of control or agency in regards to events.

> First of all, the stories that people tell are one way of reclaiming some measure of agency. No matter how buffeted one has been by events, at least one can take charge of how the story is told and, in this way, rescue oneself from passivity. To tell a story allows one to make something of experience and, thereby, of oneself (Ochberg, 1996, pp. 97–98).

The created story interweaves our identity and adaptation to life events, including health events such as injury or disability.

In this chapter, I consider the health and healing aspects of narrative from the client's perspective—how the person with a disability or illness benefits from narrative. In the next chapter (Chapter 3), a narrative approach to the clinician's role in the clinical process is discussed.

Narrative Approaches to Health and Healing

A narrative approach in many domains has developed over the last decades, including most obviously literature and communication, but extending into linguistics, psychology, and medicine. Allied health disciplines, too, have followed this move towards narrative approaches in research and clinical applications.

The roots of a narrative approach seem to be in postmodernism. Postmodernism proposes that our perception of reality is a cognitive-emotional construction, and that our experiences are filtered through individual mental schemas (Olsen, 2005). A postmodernist stance includes the position that realities are socially constructed, and social constructionism is an environment for the development of narrative approaches across a number of disciplines (Crossley, 2003). The social construction of perceived reality relies on language as both a producer of human reality and a product. These realities are organized and maintained through narrative. Since language and narrative are dynamic, this implies that realities are dynamic, and there are no essential truths (Lee, 2004).

In this view, narrative is seen as the means for coherence, to hold together our experiences, reactions, memories, and future hopes. It is also the way in which we relate to others and understand something of their own experiences, perceptions, and realities. Narrative holds a core position in considering how humans think and act in the world, and how they understand the world. The Narrative Principle is a broad view of how central narrative and narrative structures are to how humans function. It suggests that "human beings think, perceive, imagine, and make moral choices according to narrative structures" (Sarbin, 1986, p. 8).

A moment's thought demonstrates the preeminent position of narrative in our everyday lives. We wake up and tell the story of our dreams, and the story of our expectations for the day ahead; we see friends and colleagues and tell stories about finding a parking space, what leftovers we have for lunch, or the story of a challenging or interesting client we saw; we ask our clients to tell us the story of what happened to them over the weekend or why they are being seen for services; we write up the story of an evaluation or research study; we receive calls from friends or chat over the dinner table about the story of our day; and at the end of it all we entertain ourselves with a book or movie—hopefully one that has a good story!

A narrative stance assumes that we are both the creators of our own narrative and actors of the evolving story. Inherent in the narrative position are dynamics—the changeable nature of narrative as it is created in different intra- and interpersonal contexts. Thus a narrative approach both demands and accommodates change. Change is the most critical aspect of the practice of speech-language pathology; when an aspect of communication is changed from normal, we get a call, and we do our best to facilitate or induce change again, for the better.

Narrative Psychology and Narrative Therapy

A narrative approach in psychology first developed in clinical psychology and psychotherapy, but it has also become an important framework in the specialties of developmental, social, personality, and cognitive psychology. Cognitive science approaches, for example, were initially derived from an information-processing or "computer" metaphor, in which human cognition was described in terms that were analogous to those developing at the time in computer science. Similar to computers who have different kinds of memories, like RAM and disk, human memory was classified into different types, and other cognitive structures were identified within the computer metaphor. A narrative approach to cognitive science moves beyond this information processing model to a view of humans as storytellers (László, 2004; Gergen & Gergen, 1986). People create meaning in their everyday lives through stories. The narrative approach contributes an explanation of the process of how people create meaning in their everyday lives at a more global level than a description of the storage and retrieval mechanisms for information.

Other subspecialties in psychology have also embraced a narrative approach for exploring human behavioral and social phenomena. The life story can be seen as unfolding over the course of a life span. A narrative approach to development leads to the investigation of meaning during different life phases relative to storytelling. Narrative psychology has been used as a framework for reconceptualizing midlife and the "midlife crisis." It has been suggested that midlife can be thought of as a time when one's life narrative is being reconsidered; the story may or may not be going along as originally envisioned. Thus, changes to the central elements of one's life story are made and the future chapters of one's life story may be reconsidered also (Rosenberg, Rosenberg, & Farrell, 1999).

In clinical psychology and psychotherapy, narrative therapy has developed as a therapeutic technique and builds upon the dynamic aspect of narrative and its social creation (Hoshmand, 2000). Narrative therapy in clinical psychology is a process in which the client creates a self-narrative through interaction with the psychotherapist; in this case, the psychotherapist aids in the social construction of perhaps a new or alternative narrative. In pastoral or religious counseling, religious stories serve as models for an individual's conduct, and show how to relate to others appropriately and morally and how to relate to one's god (Belzen, 1996). Stories are used as mechanisms of enculturation socially and religiously; we learn how to act in a socially acceptable way by hearing the examples of stories. In religion, we may also attempt to take on important elements of a particular story as part of our own identity and self-narrative.

In narrative therapy, the psychotherapist begins with the position that the client is the protagonist in his story, and is actively acting out his own self-narrative. A key therapeutic technique in narrative therapy is narrative deconstruction, in which individuals separate the acting out of their self-narrative from their ability to produce a narrative. The separation of their actions from their narrative should engender a sense of agency and empowerment that can facilitate change. Once the self-narrative is objectified, the individual is able to consider alternatives in the narrative and exercise choices and effect change (Crossley, 2000).

The initial views of memory in a traditional information-processing approach were of memory as a process that took in information and stored it verbatim, similar to a snapshot. But as empirical evidence including neurobiological evidence has mounted, memory is now seen as a reconstruction of previous experience, and thus memory is highly dependent on the context in which the original memory was experienced and stored. A social constructionist, narrative twist to a view of memory is that memories are constructed based on overarching narrative schemas. Memories also can change somewhat based on the context in which they are recreated, in addition to the context in which they were originally stored. Memory is a dynamic reconstruction of previous experience and our memory of a particular event will alter depending on our conversational partner, the overall conversation topic, and other contextual aspects of the interaction. Thus memories can be changed; they are malleable in regards to current context and current demands for reconstruction (Olsen, 2005). Through narrative deconstruction, individuals can willfully change the meaning and content of past experience. One potential goal of narrative therapy is to alter memories of events that contribute to a current self-narrative, and create a new, more healthful or desirable self-narrative.

Narrative therapy is seen as a means of changing one's self-narrative and, by doing so, changing behaviors. Once a different story is envisioned, the individual acts out that story by engaging in various behaviors, some of which may be new or modified. As an extreme case example, narratives of ex-convicts who have been successfully reintegrated into a crime-free life show themes of changing the life story to reflect the new behaviors (Maruna, 1997).

Narrative has infused itself into the formal thinking of many disciplines. Psychology has long been closely linked with speech-language pathology; both fields have both clinical and experimental domains. Narrative psychology offers a developmental and social view of human behavior and can be applied in clinical procedures. Thus a narrative approach can be embraced for its conceptual power as well as its potential curative effects. The latter are especially relevant for speech-language pathologists and their clients who are dealing with disability, injury, or illness.

Health and Expressive Writing

Narrative therapy as practiced by clinical psychologists and other mental health professionals is a counseling process in which the psychotherapist facilitates the creation of a more desirable self-narrative as a means of coping with current problems or improving oneself. Another narrative technique that produces benefits to health is expressive writing.

The most frequently-cited research linking expressive writing and health is the work of Pennebaker and colleagues (Pennebaker, 1997; 2002). The Pennebaker paradigm involves having participants write about their traumatic or emotional experiences for 15 to 30 minutes per day for 3 to 5 consecutive days as a therapeutic writing activity. Research investigating the effects of this form of therapeutic writing typically compares writing about anxiety-producing or emotional events to writing about emotionally neutral topics such as mundane daily events.

Expressive writing can produce positive health and behavioral outcomes (Frisini, Borod, & Lepore, 2004; Lepore & Smyth, 2002; Pennebaker & Graybeal, 2001). Writing in this way about emotional experiences is linked to fewer physician visits 2 to 14 months after the expressive writing experience. This kind of expressive writing is also linked to improved immune system functioning, even in HIV-infected patients (Petrie, Fontanilla, Thomas, Booth, & Pennebaker, 2004). Finally, behavioral outcomes such as an increased likelihood of finding a new job after being laid off and improved grades among college students have also been related to participation in such a writing experience.

The concept underlying the relationship between expressive writing about traumatic events and health is the importance of mapping language and specific words to one's traumatic experiences, including experienced emotions. It is hypothesized that putting emotional experiences into words requires imposing a particular structure—a narrative structure—on the experience, thus assigning and creating meaning.

In their work, Pennebaker and colleagues have identified two critical components to the relationship between expressive writing and health. First, the account of the traumatic experience must be in the form of a story (Pennebaker & Seagal, 1999). The story very likely will evolve from a collection of disjointed perceptions to a coherent narrative as it is retold and repeated. The second critical element is verbal labeling of emotions. Words must be assigned to emotional experiences as the traumatic event is described.

The cognitive change hypothesis has been repeatedly observed within a series of studies investigating the outcomes of writing about emotionally upsetting events. The cognitive change hypothesis suggests that the more frequent usage of particular vocabulary items over the course of an expressive writing intervention is related to a greater developing sense of meaning and coherence in thinking about the traumatic event. Vocabulary usage in written samples is analyzed and categorized. Two important categories of vocabulary items are words reflecting insight and causality. Insight is suggested in words such as *realize*, *see*, and *understand*. The causality vocabulary category includes items such as *because*, *infer*, and *thus*. An increase in the use of insight and causation words from the first writing session to the last writing session is related to fewer doctor visits, improved immune functioning, and positive lifestyle changes such as higher grades (Pennebaker, Mayne, & Francis, 1997).

In addition to facilitating the generation of coherence and meaning, expressive writing is a way of forming a vision of a different future. Optimists, by definition, tend to have a positive outlook on potential future events, and are also reported as being more compliant with medical regimens. Pessimists are less likely to be compliant with regimens. Among a group of HIV-infected women, those women who were more pessimistic became more optimistic in their view of the future after a writing intervention that required the participants to write about a positive future. On the contrary, women who were more optimistic tended to show the opposite effect (Mann, 2001). At least for the more pessimistic participants, then, a writing intervention could lead to greater treatment compliance.

Health and Narrative in Self-Help Groups

Narratives can occur in the one-to-one context of a psychotherapy session or in the one-to-one context of writing when only the clinician or experimenter is going to read the writing. In both of these cases, the participant is telling his or her story to a listener who is a presumed expert or authority but has not necessarily experienced the issue under discussion. In contrast, narratives that are produced in a self-help group are constructed by the individual in the context of peers who are grappling with similar issues and challenges (Bulow, 2004). Stories are central to any self-help group.

The quintessential example of stories and self-help groups comes from the well-known organization, Alcoholics Anonymous (AA). The routine of standing in front of a group of others facing a similar problem and telling one's story has become so familiar that the format is often adapted for jokes. It is generally accepted that attendance and participation in AA meetings increases the likelihood of abstaining from alcohol abuse, and the narrative structure of the meetings has been attributed to this self-help group's success (Cercle, 2002). The story shared by an individual at such a meeting helps that individual to create meaning, a way of coping with past losses, and a hopeful outlook for the future. Those listening to an individual's story in such a meeting are given the opportunity to project themselves into that individual's story and reflect on their own circumstances.

Other kinds of self-help or support groups have also successfully incorporated a more specific narrative approach. For example, a support group for stepmothers provided a means of comparing and contrasting stepmothers' stories, and broad similarities were identified across stories, generating four major themes or story outlines about stepmothers' circumstances in role negotiation. This provides the individual with a way of identifying with a group and decreasing a sense of isolation. At the same time, individual differences can be shared through stories that preserve the individual's sense of self (Jones, 2004).

In addition to the more familiar sharing of spoken personal stories in a support group context, therapeutic writing can be employed in a group format as well. In group sessions, individuals write their own story, which is then shared with a partner and then can be read to the entire group. Therapeutic writing in a group format enhances emotional catharsis, self-knowledge, coping strategies, and understanding others (Chandler, 2002).

Group sessions and support groups for people with communication disorders often provide an opportunity to share each individual's story in some way. Just as it does in other support groups, this reduces a sense of isolation because clients begin to see the commonalities between their experiences and the experiences of others with the same communication disorder. At the same time, it enables the individual participant to proclaim her own uniqueness in a supportive setting.

Both narrative psychotherapy and expressive writing, as they occur in one-to-one settings, have been linked to positive health outcomes. Support group attendance is typically linked with behavioral outcomes, particularly when the support group is focused on behavior change, like AA. But other types of support groups, like support groups for caregivers of chronically ill individuals, have measured other kinds of outcomes. Psychoeducational groups for caregivers of spouses with Alzheimer's dementia, for example, have been shown to increase the length of time that the patient could be cared for at home, thus reducing health care costs by decreasing length of time in an institution. Furthermore, attendance at caregiver support groups tends to decrease health care visits and physical complaints on the part of the caregiver (Mittelman et al., 1994; Schulz, Williamson, & Morycz, 1993). This suggests that there are likely important similar outcomes that could be investigated for support groups of people with communication disorders and/or their caregivers. Frequency of health care visits, reports of physical symptomatology, and immune system functioning are potential physical health outcomes that could be added to the potential psychological health benefits of support groups.

Literature and Healing

Reading stories or listening to others' stories is also a way in which we begin the process of meaning-making. We identify with a character in a story and more readily imagine ourselves in that situation. Thus, reading personal narratives of others who have experienced a similar illness or disability can also facilitate change. Reading literature that includes a character with which the individual can identify based on certain common attributes, or stories in which predominant themes meet the emotional needs of the client, can provide a window to processing emotional reactions and develop coping mechanisms. Bibliotherapy and poetry therapy are examples of realms in which participating in creative writing—reading and writing—are seen to produce positive psychological benefits for those dealing with trauma or illness (Silverberg, 2003).

When the character's predicament is similar to our own, and we are in an emotionally vulnerable state, it is possible for the story to be too potent for our emotional capacity at that time. Berman (2001) notes this phenomenon in classroom teaching, in which he observes the exceptional vulnerability of three undergraduates as they were reading assigned literary pieces as part of a college course. He discusses the possibility of "risky reading" in which the assigned piece confronts issues of death, illness, or other emotionally powerful experiences, and how this kind of reading could put a particularly vulnerable student at risk. This observation underscores the potential power of literary reading as a form of emotional processing.

Bibliotherapy and its potential applications in speech-language pathology are discussed further in Chapter 15.

Benefits of Narrative to Health and Healing

When illness or disability strikes, new life behaviors may need to be learned and integrated into one's everyday routine. But even before new behavior patterns, routines, or habits are identified, the initial trauma of the onset of illness must be coped with emotionally and the long-term consequences grappled with. Narrative can be a way to re-gather coherence in one's life after trauma such as serious illness, injury, or onset or identification of disability.

General Benefits of Narrative after Illness

Initial onset of disability is a time of emotional turmoil, and has been characterized as a disruption of one's life narrative. The individual who is still in the midst of absorbing the trauma may be upset when considering his or her previous life before the trauma, and equally upset when contemplating an undefined and unpredictable future.

At this point there is a lack of temporal and emotional distance between the trauma and the individual, so telling one's life narrative during such a period could be distressing.

As time passes and coping develops, telling one's life story may have a few potential benefits. First, creating a life narrative after onset of disability may help the individual to obtain cohesion between past life events and the present circumstances. The narrative of the present may slowly be able to accommodate the existence of the disability. As this occurs, envisioning future plans and goals may be facilitated, as a coherent narrative that bridges all events through time develops.

The linkages between onset of disability and the development of a life narrative may of course be related to age and human development. For example, older adults who experience stroke and consequent disability do not necessarily experience a disruption in life narrative. In one study, narratives of individuals with stroke were analyzed and the researchers found that biographical flow was more consistent in the narratives than biographical disruption (Faircloth, Boylstein, Young, & Gubrium, 2004). Understanding patients' perspectives of their lives and how illnesses or disabilities fit into them may lead to more effective or at least more cohesive interventions.

The nature of life narratives and how these are linked to disability may have more to do with positive or negative attitude, perhaps, than with the nature of the illness or trauma. For example, life stories were collected from 107 seniors who had chronic illness and were living in the community (Montbriand, 2004). Those seniors who had more optimistic perceptions were less likely to connect their life experiences with current illnesses. Those individuals with more pessimistic views were more likely to link their life experiences with their present illness, and were also more likely to recall past abuses and coping with past abuse. The tone of the individual's life narrative seems to persist through disabling events to older age.

Younger adults will perhaps experience more disruption to the life narrative, possibly because there is a greater difference between expectations for illness and disability at a young age than there is at an older age (Baltes, 2003). These sociocultural expectations for what kinds of life events are most likely to occur at particular ages are infused into the narrative schema of each individual, and are part of the cultural context in which they are created.

Children living with disabilities will learn about typical expectations, and as they develop, they may begin to see the differences between typical sociocultural expectations and their own potential life narratives. The child with a disability, like every other individual, will interpret individual differences from typical expectations either positively or negatively.

A second potential benefit of telling one's life story after illness or trauma is its potential to reduce a sense of isolation. Narration brings experiences into consciousness, and sharing one's narrative may decrease isolation and alienation. This is most commonly accomplished through the sharing of life narratives in the context of a support group. Individuals who have sustained a communication disability traumatically may often repeat the narrative of their illness to clinicians, other patients, friends, and family. The repetition of the illness events may serve in part as an effort to integrate illness events into one's life narrative, to make sense of past life events with current circumstances, and to decrease isolation by seeking out empathy and understanding.

Third, creation of a narrative during a period of accommodation to disability may enable an individual to incorporate his or her identity with new health behaviors (Rosenthal, 2003). Individuals living with a disability are likely to need to take medication, do their exercises, practice their speech homework, or develop new or alternative means of accomplishing everyday tasks. When these new behaviors need to be performed over the long term, the individual will need to stop thinking of them as a temporary reaction to illness and start thinking of these behaviors as part of their identity.

Our ability to adhere to new health behaviors is influenced by narratives that we engage in with ourselves and with others. A common health behavior change is to integrate exercise into one's lifestyle. Adherence to such a new health regimen seems to be dependent on the presence of self-narratives and the narratives that are shared with support persons. These narratives must reflect the integration of the exercise regimen into one's identity in order for the new behavior to endure (McGannon, 2002). Our self-narrative must be changed to accommodate a desired new behavior.

Finally, narration may decrease the effects of stress associated with illness or injury onset. For example, narrative-expressive therapy has been used to combat the effects of stress stemming from dealing with cancer, the onset of which has been described as a traumatic event (Petersen, Bull, Probst, Dettinger, & Detwiler, 2005). It has been reported that 13% of cancer patients experience post-traumatic stress disorder. A narrative approach aids patients dealing with cancer to construct meaning, decrease stress, and adapt to their current circumstances. It is possible that narrative therapy could reduce stress effects in other traumatic-onset conditions, as well.

Narrative can be construed as a way in which we develop our own identity. Because of the dynamic aspect of narrative, it can be identified as a source for behavior change, as it is in narrative therapy. Narratives can be analyzed for showing how individuals accommodate to health changes, and how new behaviors including health behaviors are assimilated into one's everyday life and therefore one's identity.

Physical and Psychological Outcomes Associated with Narratives

Narratives have been linked to a variety of physical and psychological outcomes in various contexts and with a variety of clinical populations. Some of these outcomes have been investigated in certain contexts in speech-language pathology, and others have not. Considering the linkages between narratives and health outcomes in other disciplines might prove fruitful for additional investigation in specialty areas of speech-language pathology.

Decreased frequency of self-reported physical symptoms has been linked to expressive writing interventions and support group participation. Another interesting and important physical health outcome that has been linked to narration is frequency of medical visits. In this case, the frequency of health care contacts is counted for a period of time before a narrative intervention and for a similar amount of time after an intervention. This is an observable measure that relates not only to the individual's welfare but also to health care costs; accessing the system less reduces the overall burden on the health care system. In some studies, specific disease-related immune functions have been monitored as a reaction to writing about a traumatic or anxiety-producing event. Improved immune system functioning has been linked to writing about emotionally traumatic events, even among those with immune disorders such as Epstein-Barr or HIV.

Psychological and emotional outcomes that have been positively related to narrative writing include perceived life satisfaction, measures of positive and negative affect, mood, self-reported anxiety, optimism, and depression. Furthermore, narrative interventions have been most productively linked to measures of adaptation and adjustment, including adjustment to illness and adjustment to typical life changes such as college adjustment.

Writing about anxiety-producing events as an intervention has not consistently produced outcomes in all contexts, however. For example, adding expressive writing to an office-based intervention for smoking cessation did not seem to enhance the effect of the behavioral program (Ames, Patten, & Offord, 2005). No differences in psychological outcomes have been observed between groups of children of divorce who write narratives about trauma or stress compared to those who write about non-emotional topics (Graybeal, 2004), nor among children of alcoholics (Gallant & Lafreniere, 2003). An expressive writing intervention did not produce measurable effects in the lung functioning of asthmatics (Harris, 2004), nor is it superior to time management for producing positive outcomes among adults with hypertension (Beckwith, 2003). Writing about suicidal thoughts did not produce the kinds of positive benefits hoped for, either; participants reported fewer automatic negative thoughts but also reported more frequent health center appointments (Kovac & Range, 2002). Thus, narrative in general and expressive writing in particular are certainly not a panacea that routinely produce multiple physical and psychological benefits.

There is clearly a complex set of relationships between personality variables including optimism/pessimism, narrative intervention, and physical or psychological outcomes. Overall, the most robust finding across multiple studies is the link between narration and psychological measures of coping. Coping successfully may lead to improved general health, decreasing medical visits, and improving immune functioning. At present, this seems the most promising avenue for investigating the potential health benefits of narration in all of its forms—narrative therapy, expressive writing, self-help groups, and participation in creative literature.

STUDY/DISCUSSION QUESTIONS AND ACTIVITIES

1. Make a list of literature or poetry that you have read and enjoyed, and that has been particularly meaningful to you. Reflect on what themes in these pieces resonate most with your personal qualities or character. How does this relate to how you practice as a speech-language pathologist?
2. If possible, consider how clients present their stories about their communication to you over time. How do their stories change as they grow older? As time passes?
3. Participate in a support group of some type. Observe the kinds of narratives that occur spontaneously between the group members.

Narrative-Based Practice

OVERVIEW

The purpose of this chapter is to describe the uses and applications of a narrative-based approach to practice in speech-language pathology. Narrative-based practice presents a holistic view of all aspects of practice and is complementary to evidence-based practice. Narrative approaches accommodate clinical expertise and provide a means to coherently integrate general conclusions drawn from evidence and individual circumstances and exceptions that are the domain of clinical expertise.

LEARNING OBJECTIVES

At the end of this chapter, the reader will be able to:

1. Contrast the contribution of evidence-based practice with the potential contribution of narrative-based practice.

2. Explain how evidence-based practice and narrative work together.

Narrative-Based Medicine, Narrative-Based Practice

Evidence-based practice, based on the initial movement in evidence-based medicine, has become part and parcel of our practice in speech-language pathology, as in all other health-related disciplines. Evidence-based practice is a process by which we ask an answerable clinical question, gather the relevant scientific evidence, and weigh that evidence systematically and statistically if possible to derive a conclusion about the best possible practice approach for our clinical question. The general goal of evidence-based practice is to come to general conclusions that may be applied across individual cases; the approach is specifically designed to minimize the influence of individual characteristics and circumstances. Such an approach is critical to clinical practice. If we cannot make general conclusions about what the most effective approach will be on average, we put ourselves in the position of reinventing a clinical approach for each new case. This is not only inefficient, but also counter to human nature. Humans are designed to find commonalities, make generalizations, and then pay attention to novelty or differences.

The ability to efficiently make generalizations is counterbalanced by how difference from the expected generality draws our attention. Narrative-based medicine highlights individual aspects of the experience of being ill and encountering the health service system. Narrative-based medicine is an approach that has its roots in the narrative principle (see Chapter 2), the assumption that narrative is central to how humans think and behave. In narrative-based medicine, narrative is viewed as a bridge between the clinician and the patient; clinicians communicate with other clinicians via narrative, clinicians and patients construct narratives together, and patients narrate together (Greenhalgh & Hurwitz, 1998). Narrative-based medicine has been described as the embedding of the body and its illnesses into the life story of the person (Clark, 2005).

A narrative perspective of the clinical process emphasizes dialogue and the social construction of the experience of illness and health within the health service system (Hatem & Rider, 2004).

Narrative provides a means to understand the holistic complexities of individuals, who are the subject of medicine. The emotional, psychological, and spiritual aspects of an individual are interwoven with the physical, and a change in one impinges on the others. Bringing narrative into the medical and health realms emphasizes a holistic approach to communication between clinicians and clients and an appreciation of the effects of medical care on the whole person (Bolton, 2005).

So, just as the principles of evidence-based medicine have been translated to evidence-based practice in speech-language pathology, I am proposing that the principles of narrative-based medicine be translated to narrative-based practice in speech-language pathology. Both evidence-based practice and narrative-based practice should happily coexist. Based on the former we derive general practice guidelines, but the latter provides a framework in which we can explore individual experiences, consider individual circumstances, and investigate the psychological and emotional aspects of the clinical process that are difficult to quantify and generalize.

In a social constructionist view, language is considered both a producer and a product of human reality. A narrative-based approach, with its roots in social constructionism, can be said to view narrative as both a producer and a product of individual and social experience. Greenhalgh and Hurwitz, in the introductory chapter of their 1998 book entitled *Narrative-Based Medicine*, describe the benefits and rationale for studying narrative in the medical context. The diagnostic, therapeutic, and educational components of the clinician-patient interaction can be served by a narrative approach. The education of other professionals and the pursuit of new knowledge in clinically-oriented research can also benefit from a narrative framework. In each aspect of traditional medical care, narrative is both a producer and a product within the health service encounter.

In the diagnostic segment of a clinician-client interaction, the patient's narrative may provide clues that will aid the clinician to more efficiently arrive at an appropriate diagnosis. Take, for example, the case of a patient with multiple health concerns who, during his initial description of his presenting problem, frequently mentions his role as caregiver for his parents. The patient also repeatedly notes that his mother had a stroke and this is increasing his care burden. In the physician-patient encounter reported by Beach (2005), these psychosocial concerns as raised by the patient were overlooked in favor of a more traditional analysis of the specific physical symptoms. Psychosocial concerns that may be root causes or critical contributors to health concerns may be ignored in traditional medical encounters. Attention to the whole narrative that a patient offers may suggest some alternative ways of dealing with these neglected but perhaps primary themes in a patient's life. A narrative approach to diagnostics also facilitates understanding between the clinician and the client, provides a glimpse into the patient's illness experience, and allows co-construction of meaning between the clinician and the client. These reasons underlie the current use of narrative in responsive nursing evaluations (Abma & Widdershoven, 2005).

During the therapeutic portion of a clinical interaction, narratives may suggest particular or alternative treatment modalities. Narratives facilitate a holistic view of the patient and the treatment. Narrative construction may in and of itself be therapeutic as it allows the patient to create meaning from experiences, reduce stress, and decrease a sense of isolation.

A narrative approach to education and professional training specifically enhances the development of clinical communication skills, empathy, and sensitivity in the developing clinician (Bleakley, 2005). Teaching clinicians to "think in stories" facilitates more holistic and integrative processing of clinical information. Otherwise, purely scientific processing of case-based information tends to produce analytic thinking that leads to decontextualized categorization.

Expertise in the Clinical Process

The expertise of the individual clinician is a critical element of the clinical process and successful outcomes. Expertise is an important component in the process of evidence-based practice (EBP; Sackett, Rosenberg, Gray, Haynes, & Richardson, 1996; Sackett, Straus,

Richardson, Rosenberg, & Haynes, 2000). Most of the attention and discussion on EBP is focused on the availability of clinical evidence, and the effective analysis of the weight of the evidence. The scientific evidence must be weighed, however, with sharp, ethical clinical judgment. The development of clinical judgment and expertise is a growing concern and area of study. It is argued that narrative approaches have much to contribute to the development of clinical expertise and to the use of evidence in practice.

Definition of Expertise

There are a variety of conceptual and theoretical frameworks for expertise and its development. Farrington-Darby & Wilson (2006) compare three approaches to defining expertise that are representative of different fields of study. In a more typical cognitive science approach (Chi, Glaser, & Farr, 1988), experts are described as individuals who excel in their own specialty and who can identify large meaningful patterns among a set of small details. Experts have also been described as those who can break down a large problem into smaller steps, using a "divide and conquer" strategy (Shanteau, 1992). Experts are fast and can perform in their area of domain quickly with few mistakes. Experts also demonstrate superior memory performance in their area of specialty. Experts spend time analyzing a problem qualitatively and exercise strong self-monitoring abilities. These characteristics seem to be accompanied by good communication skills in their domain and a corresponding knowledge about resources to draw on for assistance when needed.

This general description of expertise corresponds to current approaches to expertise and its development in the profession of speech-language pathology (Guilford, Graham, & Scheuerle, 2007). In the O'Sullivan and Doutis (1994) model described by Guilford and colleagues, expertise in many domains including speech-language pathology can be characterized by 12 characteristics. The first two characteristics of experts are an increase in the accuracy and ease with which experts can solve problems in their domain. Experts initially acquired knowledge via weak methods, but ultimately develop the ability to perceive important patterns within their domain, respond automatically, and remember pertinent information in a superior manner. With specific goals and practice, expertise can be developed within the specific domain or profession. Experts search through data forward rather than backward from goals while solving domain-specific problems. Experts perform consistently; their performance can be predicted from declared rules or guidelines. Fortunately, once aspects of expertise in any particular domain are defined, these practices can be taught to develop expertise among novices.

Initial or ongoing training can be formulated in such a way to facilitate the development of expertise starting at the novice stage. Arts, Gijselaers, and Segers (2006) compared the results of training students using a traditional problem-based learning approach (PBL) to a refined problem-based learning technique. The refined design included problem descriptions that were not preanalyzed, ill-structured information rather than structured information presentation, and multimedia format of information. Students in the refined design were expected to brainstorm on all aspects of the case and the possible solution, and assigned themselves roles for addressing the problem. Students who participated in the refined version of PBL used more domain-specific concepts, tended to use more inductive reasoning, and produced diagnostic conclusions and solutions of higher quality than the students who participated in traditional PBL. The nature of the reasoning demonstrated by the students in the refined PBL group, the use of knowledge, and the generation of higher quality outputs are consistent with the development of expertise. These refined procedures—such as presenting information in more naturalistic, "messy" ways—facilitated the development of these characteristics among novices.

Practice or time-on-task is a consistently identified component in the development of expertise. The literature on expertise suggests the "10,000 hour" rule, in which expertise in any given domain requires 10,000 hours of practice or time-on-task (Ericsson, Krampe, & Tesch-Romer, 1993). It has even been argued that child prodigies very likely conform to this general observation; in spite of Mozart's young age at the time of his first composition, it is possible that he had put in his 10,000 hours. For a speech-language pathologist, the 10,000 hour rule implies that 250 work weeks (40 hours per week) are necessary to achieve the 10,000 hours, and this translates to about 5 years of experience (assuming a 48-week work year). It is probably not surprising that many job-related or profession-related definitions of expert require a minimum of 3, 5, or even 7 years' experience.

The accumulation of expert skills requires time and experience; thus, experts are to be found among those professionals who have some number of years of experience in their area of practice. Years of experience alone, however, does not necessarily yield expertise. According to the often used definitions of expertise, these years of experience must have resulted in fast, accurate performance in which both pattern recognition and decomposition skills are deployed. Experts have also developed a network of resources—published works, unpublished works, and knowledge about how to contact other experts—that results in the successful completion of targeted tasks.

In speech-language pathology in the United States we recognize expertise through specialty recognition. In neurogenics, board certification by the Academy of Neurologic Communication Disorders & Sciences requires the demonstration of content knowledge through successful completion of a multiple-choice exam, as well as demonstration of highly developed procedural abilities and knowledge through a written case presentation. Initiation of the pursuit of specialty recognition is preceded by a minimum requirement of number of years of professional experience. Similar demonstrations of experience, declarative knowledge, and procedural knowledge are required for specialty recognition through one of ASHA's Special Interest Divisions, such as Fluency and Dysphagia.

In some disciplines, expertise is defined primarily based on outcomes or arrival at a successful solution to a problem. In other disciplines, the study of expertise is focused on the process used by experts to tackle problems (Farrington-Darby & Wilson, 2006). A process view of expertise is likely to contribute most to a discussion of its development in speech-language pathology, and to map on to the process of evidence-based practice, as well.

Expertise and Evidence-Based Practice

EBP is the integration of "individual clinical expertise with the best available external clinical evidence from systematic research" (Sackett, et al., 1996). It derives from the position that expert opinion alone is not sufficient for appropriate clinical decision-making. EBP takes the stance that treatments can produce harm, and therefore ethical, expert practice must rely on the application and implementation of best practices as demonstrated by weighty clinical evidence.

It does bear noting, however, that the first part of Sackett et al.'s (1996) classic definition is "individual clinical expertise." Thus the foundation or frame for integrating evidence into practice still must be the expert clinician.

The first step in incorporating EBP into an ethical, expert practice is to be familiar with and to weigh the scientific evidence for the treatment of a particular disorder (see, for example, Johnson, 2006). Thus, the expert clinician must continuously monitor the developing research in his typical areas of practice. This can be accomplished by regularly attending workshops and conferences that offer scientific updates on treatment techniques. Monitoring journals and publications, including on-line resources, is another important way to keep abreast of scientific advances in treatment. Finally, periodic searches of particular scientific resources, easily accomplished on-line, are also a way for the expert clinician to maintain contact with the scientific treatment literature.

Pursuing these techniques will expose the clinician to a variety of types of scientific evidence. But following single studies as they are published is not the equivalent of knowing the weight of all of the evidence in a particular practice area taken together. An important tenet of EBP is to weigh the evidence, and consider the type of evidence that is available for any given treatment. If I find a new treatment that sounds "just right" for the client who is currently challenging my clinical skills and knowledge, is the one study I've found a sufficient base from which I can reasonably expect benefit?

The process of weighing the evidence is typically described in terms of analyzing the research designs, reliability, and validity of studies as well as the number of studies of high quality that report a particular outcome. The American Speech-Language-Hearing Association has characterized different types of experimental studies in four levels of evidence (ASHA, 2005), adapted from the Scottish Intercollegiate Guideline Network. The highest level of evidence (Level I) in this guideline is the randomized controlled trial. When some number of these randomized controlled trial studies have been completed for a particular treatment or disorder area, it is possible to conduct a meta-analysis of the studies. A meta-analysis is a technique that allows the results of several studies to be statistically analyzed (Robey & Dalebout, 1998). The result demonstrates the weight of the evidence across several studies in favor of or against a particular treatment.

Among the lower levels of evidence are studies that do not include randomization, single-subject designs, correlational and case studies (Levels II and III). Finally, the clinical experience of respected authorities in a given specialization can be taken as the weakest form of evidence (Level IV).

From this system are derived terms that can be used to describe classes of treatments (ASHA, 2004). Standards are accepted principles of patient care based on a high degree of certainty and Level I or strong Level II evidence. Guidelines reflect a moderate degree of certainty, are not fixed protocols or rigid treatment rules, and are typically based on Level II evidence. Golper (2001, pp. x) describes practice guidelines as "explicit descriptions of how patients should be evaluated and treated," and their purpose is to "improve and assure the quality of care by reducing unacceptable variation in its provision." Organized, systematic reviews are undertaken and evaluated against established criteria to produce practice guidelines. The products of these reviews are published findings that summarize the weight of published evidence for any particular treatment or assessment that can be used by clinicians (Frattali et al., 2003). Treatments or assessments that are only supported by limited evidence or conflicting studies should only be considered as treatment options.

For example, a Cochrane review is available for speech and language treatment for children and adolescents with primary speech and language delay/disorder (Law, Garrett, & Nye, 2004). The review considered the results of 25 randomized controlled trials after a systematic and exhaustive search of the literature. The results of the meta-analysis suggested that treatment for children with phonological and vocabulary difficulties is effective, but there was less evidence for the effectiveness of treatment for children with receptive language difficulties. There were also only mixed results for the effectiveness of intervention for syntactic impairments. There was no difference in the effectiveness of treatment administered individually or in groups, but the incorporation of normal language peers into the intervention had a positive effect, as determined by results across the 25 studies. These broad conclusions that are based on analysis of 25 well-designed studies can be persuasive evidence to parents, practitioners of other disciplines, or third-party payers about the usefulness of certain speech-language pathology services. A report such as this Cochrane review also highlights areas in which additional clinical research is needed. In this case, more research is needed for treatment for receptive and syntactical disorders.

These broad conclusions are insufficient for tackling all of the individual-specific considerations for any given client who walks through your door. Expertise—not just the acquisition of knowledge but the development of its appropriate use and the reasoning and social skills required for its use—plays a fundamental role in the ability of clinicians to implement appropriately any identified practice guideline. Expertise is often developed through narrative and probably also carried out through narrative.

Implementation of any particular practice guideline is dependent on the ability of the clinician to match the guideline to an individual case (typically not described in the actual guideline); inferential thinking and abstraction are required on the part of the clinician to perform this task. Then, given the client's resources, client's environment, and the clinical resources, the clinician must determine whether adherence to a recommended treatment or practice is feasible or whether it is likely to produce the desired outcome. This requires the clinician to reason forward through the unstructured details available and to identify critical informational elements that she or he must have in order to pursue appropriate actions for the client. Implementation of practice guidelines, then, is highly dependent on clinical expertise.

At every step along an evidence-based practice path, the clinician's judgment, reasoning skills, speed of processing relevant information, pattern identification of relevant information, and other characteristics of expertise are relied on. The more we think about evidence-based practice, the more we realize that the scientific evidence—while critical—is a relatively small piece of the clinical process. What is ever-present at every step in the process is the expertise of the clinician.

Practice guidelines, even when appropriate and possible to implement, are only as predictive as the reliability with which the clinician implements them. How much difference can seemingly small changes in implementation really make to the outcome of a treatment program? A study investigating outcomes of social skills training for students with moderate to severe disabilities provides an example (McEvoy, Shores, Wehby, Johnson, & Fox, 1990). After the study on outcomes of social skills training was completed, the researchers divided the special education teachers who had participated in the study into two groups: those teachers with the highest treatment integrity (or reliability with which the independent variable or treatment was implemented) and those with the lowest treatment integrity. Students whose teachers were in the high treatment integrity group had superior outcomes to those students taught by teachers with low treatment integrity.

In another education-related example, students' performance in a math instructional program was measured under conditions of complete and accurate implementation and lower levels of integrity (Noell, Gresham, & Gansle, 2002). The math instruction program protocol included systematic prompts to the students to use specified strategies. The study compared the performance of students when they received the prompts called for in the program 100% of the time, 67% of the time, and 33% of the time, to mimic inconsistent or partial implementation. Students performed significantly better when they received the instructional program with 100% treatment integrity.

When we base our clinical decision-making processes on scientific evidence first, then we must be willing to implement a specific treatment program in the same way in which it originally demonstrated its effectiveness. If treatments are not administered in the way in which they were used during the accumulation of the evidence, then they might be null and void. On the other hand, of course, implementation of a procedure according to its original standard could produce unusual or unexpected reactions in an individual, and the clinician must be alert to these possibilities as well. So, again, the expertise of the clinician is critical.

It has only been about 15 years since the principles of evidence-based practice have become more prevalent and integrated into all aspects of health care. The production of treatment research and the generation of practice guidelines take years to accomplish. It is not surprising, then, that in spite of our best professional efforts we do not yet have practice guidelines for all of the disorder categories in speech-language pathology. Nor do we have yet an evidentiary base that provides guidance under unusual circumstances. Where the foundation of the scientific evidence comes to an end for a particular treatment or disorder, the clinician's expertise must take over in the clinical decision-making process.

There are two broad categories in which the clinician's expertise plays a prominent role in clinical management decisions (Hinckley, 2007). First, there may be situations which appear to be subject to available evidence, but individual characteristics or circumstances present a potential challenge to the available scientific base. Second, there may be clinical problems for which there is very little scientific evidence available.

Although it is convenient to think about the two kinds of clinical situations in which clinical expertise will play a prominent role, it may be misleading. To describe clinical expertise as playing a primary role when the evidence fails us is to take the position that the evidence is primary in the clinical decision-making process. This is probably false; clinical expertise is the soil in which evidence grows and is harvested. It is more realistic and more productive to consider how clinical expertise is the filter through which studies are designed, conclusions are made, individual patients are greeted, their problems identified, treatments considered and implemented, and outcomes measured.

Narrative, Expertise, and Evidence-Based Practice

The broad conclusions that derive from quantitative approaches are critical for many contexts, especially for policy development. But every clinician knows that the knowledge of general practice guidelines or other generalized conclusions about assessment or treatment may not be able to adequately address the individual-specific concerns of the next client who walks through the door. These individual-specific challenges and issues are best dealt with by narrative-based approaches. The clinician will first facilitate the telling of the client's own narrative, and the clinician will develop her or his own story about the client. This will be an important part of how the clinician considers appropriate courses of action for that particular client and determines how best to implement them. It can also be argued that the clinician will think about when it is appropriate to discharge clients based on whether the story of the client's pursuit of identified goals has come to a sufficient ending or not.

Clinical expertise, which has very often been accumulated in narratives, thought about in narratives, and shared in narratives, is the constant backdrop for steps in the process of evidence-based practice. We started our exploration of narrative-based practice with the idea that we "dream in narrative, daydream in narrative, remember, anticipate, hope, despair, believe, doubt, plan, revise, criticize, construct, gossip, learn, hate and love by narrative" (Hardy, 1986, p. 5). Thinking in narrative is the way in which any individual clinician will go through the steps of EBP.

The first step in EBP is to ask an answerable clinical question. A structure for asking these questions has been proposed and is widely used, following the acronym PICO. The components of this acronym stand for population (P), intervention (I), comparison (C), and outcome (O). An answerable clinical question should contain each of the elements in the question in a specific manner. The structure may be provided, but the content of the question relies on the ability of the clinician to identify key elements of the client's situation and translate them to a larger narrative that is made up of our clinical science. In narrative terms, the clinician is mapping the roles and needs of one "character" (the client) in a narrative that is about the treatment of the communication disability of lots of other people like that one client.

In the search for evidence, the clinician will systematically access common databases and sources. Yet one individual clinician may find a different set of evidence from another individual clinician. Most productive and well-done systematic reviews, for example, rely on the work of a group of scientists who collectively manage not only the quantity of sources found, but also make unique contributions to the search. Searching for evidence is a process of identifying key words that embody the general themes attributable to a question. Knowledge of the procedures that render a search effective is not sufficient to produce a useful search for clinical evidence. The clinician is identifying and finding key elements that match the story of the client in question to the larger story told in the clinical literature.

Analyzing the evidence, in narrative terms, amounts to telling a meta-narrative across studies. Researchers talk informally about the story in their data, and this is true for either quantitative or qualitative studies. Qualitative techniques can be applied to produce a meta-narrative across studies (e.g., Greenhalgh et al., 2005). Although narrative techniques are typically not explicitly acknowledged or applied when bodies of evidence are weighed, the narrative framework for information management is inherent in the process.

Finally, clinical decision-making is conducted with the analyzed evidence as one source of information. If the clinical evidence points clearly down a strongly supported path, the clinician can select that route as appropriate for the client in question. In many cases in speech-language pathology, however, there is not sufficiently strong evidence to provide clear direction for the clinician. The clinician must mix what is understood from the clinical evidence with clinical experience and expertise, along with individual considerations for that particular client. In narrative terms, this is akin to being provided with a description of three different characters—one named Evidence, another named Experience, and the third named Client. These three characters are embarking on a journey together, and it is the clinician's job to weave a tale about how the three characters manage to get along and arrive at their desired destination. It is difficult to imagine that narrative structures, narrative thinking, and narrative abilities do not play a role in the effective implementation of evidence-based practice.

Summary

A narrative-based approach offers a framework for attacking issues of clinical practice that are otherwise difficult to address. These issues include how narrative is used by clients to present problems and share their perspectives; how analysis of the clinician-client communication reveals the narrative constructed by the interaction; how narratives play a role in professional development and cohesiveness; and how narrative contributes importantly to professional and preprofessional training. The contributions of a narrative-based approach must be weaved together with conclusions from evidence to generate the most comprehensive and powerful portrayal of the clinical interaction possible, along with holistic recommendations for clinician and client behavior.

STUDY/DISCUSSION QUESTIONS AND ACTIVITIES

1. Weave a story about how you applied a practice guideline or other evidence to a particular client's case. Does the story have a happy ending?
2. Locate three resources for practice guidelines or other relevant evidence for your area of specialty.
3. Tell a story about how your personal clinical experience and expertise made a significant difference in the case of a particular client.

Section II

Fundamentals of Narratives

Narrative Methods of Inquiry

OVERVIEW

This chapter will provide an overview of narrative methodologies including their assumptions, purposes, and products. The general paradigms associated with narrative research methods are explored, and three examples of particular methodologies are described. Finally, some ethical considerations that must be confronted when conducting narrative research are raised.

LEARNING OBJECTIVES

At the end of this chapter, the reader will be able to:

1. Contrast positivist and constructionist paradigms.

2. Describe three examples of narrative research methodologies.

3. List procedures commonly associated with in-depth interviewing.

4. Discuss three ethical considerations for narrative research.

Introduction to Narrative Methodology

The study of narrative and the use of narrative as a research methodology have been active areas of study for some time now, but it is only within the last few years that narrative research has been specifically applied to domains such as the health sciences and education. Narrative research techniques cannot suit all purposes; like any other research methodology, narrative methodologies are well-suited to certain kinds of exploration and study and completely unsuitable for others. It is perhaps a sign of the sophistication of the development of research tools in the health- and education-related disciplines that a variety of research techniques can be employed to match the full range of scientific inquiry.

Generally, the job of the narrative researcher is to analyze the stories that people tell. If one takes the stance that stories are both a means and a product of sense-making for one's life and the activities and events therein, then the analysis of stories can be viewed as a powerful tool for learning about experiences and perceptions. Narrative techniques can also be employed to summarize empirical data in meaningful and useable ways.

Narrative analysts tend to analyze the form, structure, and content of the story, asking why the story was told that particular way under those circumstances. These narrative analytic techniques are generally quite familiar to speech-language pathologists, because we have long been interested in knowing whether our clients are able to understand and appropriately use narrative structures, producing the semantic-syntactic forms that are relevant to a given stimulus or task. We have also been interested in our clients' abilities to be sensitive to the listener, using appropriate pragmatic skills given the context of the narrative. Typically we are assessing these aspects of narrative under relatively structured and controlled conditions; that is, we are providing picture stimuli or suggesting a story to be retold. We do not often use personal narratives or life narratives as a task for assessing narrative abilities, nor do we often use personal narrative or life narratives formally as a source for intervention activities (but see Biddle, McCabe, & Bliss, 1996, for one exception). There are exceptions to this; of course we use personally relevant topics and activities when selecting stimulus materials or identifying functional activities to target in treatment. (For an example of using autobiographical narratives to plan, deliver, and evaluate a course for partners of adults with aphasia, see Pound, Parr, & Duchan, 2001.) But listening to our client's list of interests or life activities in response to our interviewing techniques is not the same as soliciting personal or life narratives and expanding our professional knowledge base accordingly. In this chapter, these future directions for using narrative techniques in speech-language pathology will be explored after a review of narrative methodologies.

Narrative can be analyzed by its components, such as its structure and content, or more holistically by its themes or overall message. These techniques rest on principles of qualitative methodologies, and are well-suited for addressing holistic questions about lived experience (Murray, 2003a; Murray, 2003b). The generation of a more holistic narrative from a review of extant literature can also provide a more meaningful conclusion to systematic review. In the next section, the roots and current development of narrative approaches are described along with a discussion about appropriate uses and applications. An overview and sample of narrative techniques follow.

Roots and Development of Narrative Approaches

As an approach to inquiry, narrative methods fit under the umbrella of the qualitative paradigm. Qualitative approaches derive from observational techniques of cultural anthropology, in which scientists participated in another culture and systematically noted and interpreted their observations. Such observations are often communicated in narratives; stories about particular rituals or events are offered as evidence for some general conclusion about the observed culture.

In spite of attempts to make objective observations, it became clear that all such cultural observations were made through one's own cultural lens. The recognition of the inherent, unavoidable subjectivity within the observational and participant-observation techniques of anthropology became acknowledged and ultimately embraced by qualitative researchers. In anthropology, early efforts to recognize this inherent subjectivity in observation led to narratives about the experience of doing participant-observation, and about living and being in a different culture. From these narratives was born a tradition of acknowledging and incorporating the observer's reactions into the report. "What happens within the observer must be made known . . . if the nature of what has been observed is to be understood" (Behar, 1997, p. 6). Reporting the internal experience of the observer has become a recognized necessity for appropriately interpreting the observations.

Qualitative approaches are designed to address "the essence of the social phenomenon and its meaning in the participants' lives" (Damico & Simmons-Mackie, 2003, p. 133).

> By word and by action, in subtle ways and in direct statements, [researchers] say, "I want to understand the world from your point of view. I want to know what you know in the way you know it. I want to understand the meaning of your experience, to walk in your shoes, to feel things as you feel them, to explain things as you would explain them. Will you become my teacher and help me understand?" (Spradley, 1979, p. 34).

Qualitative clinical research can help to expose and explore areas of clinical experience that are not readily addressed by quantitative methods, such as the understanding of disease and disability as a cultural construction and the appreciation of alternative models of illness and healing, including holistic models (Miller & Crabtree, 2003). "Qualitative research also recognizes that the therapeutic or healing process occurs not only in the clinical moment, but also in the everyday life between clinical events" (Miller & Crabtree, 2003, p. 405).

Qualitative approaches include a wide array of research techniques, including conversational and discourse analysis, rhetorical analyses, ethnography and ethnographic narratives. Conversational and discourse analysis are familiar creatures in the speech-language pathology landscape. Rhetorical analyses are the use of narrative structures to analyze broad themes within a set of qualitative data, such as interview data, or to explore the meta-narrative produced across a number of studies. Examples of rhetorical analyses will be discussed more in the next section of this chapter.

Ethnography has been defined in various ways (Tedlock, 2000), but the primary characteristic of ethnography is the embedding of field observations within culture (McQuiston, Parrado, Colmos-Muniz, & Bustillo Martinez, 2005). Ethnographic methods emphasize participant-observation, in which the observer becomes an active participant in the culture being studied. Participant-observation is distinct from traditional observational techniques in which the researcher separates him- or herself from the participants in the topic of study; in participant-observation the observer becomes a full-fledged member of the group of interest. Research tools within ethnography include a variety of interviewing techniques, focus groups, and other interactions in which individuals share their particular views or experiences in a systematic, reciprocal fashion with the investigator. Ethnographic methods are particularly well-suited to exploring the "insider" view of a particular culture or experience. Narrative ethnography, in particular, is a term that refers to ethnographic approaches that emphasize the dialogue between participants and observers (McQuiston et al, 2005).

Narrative approaches find roots in several disciplines, including linguistics, literature, communication, and anthropology, extending from the humanities into the social and behavioral sciences. Narrative approaches can include interviewing and may also rely heavily on interaction between the participants and the observer. Narrative ethnography rests on story-making and storytelling; in some forms of narrative ethnography, such as autoethnography, self-reflection and narrative provide the source of dialogue, observation, and reporting.

Although qualitative research approaches are not new to speech-language pathology, they have as yet been less frequently applied to questions of clinical practice in our field than in many other disciplines (Damico & Simmons-Mackie, 2003). In other domains that are strongly related to speech-language pathology, qualitative approaches and narrative methods in particular are much more fully evolved and acknowledged. While in speech-language pathology we are still in the early stages of identifying appropriate applications and accepting qualitative research methods, other fields have passed this stage and have simply pressed on with accepting and performing qualitative and ethnographic work. Freeman (2001) describes this development from an early phase of recognition to a simple acceptance of narrative methods:

> . . . narrative inquiry has reached what might be called a "post-polemical" phase. By this I mean that most of those working in the area of narrative for some time are generally less concerned to indict the status quo, particularly in its positivistic form, than was once the case. Moreover, they are less concerned to defend their own work, to argue for its right to exist or its superiority over traditional social science approaches. Rather than proposing to do the desired work or proclaiming the need for such work, it is simply being done, constructively and vigorously. In part, this is because the cause of critique, important though it surely is, can sometimes get old; there is just so much time and energy to be devoted essentially to negation (p. 283).

In some fields related to speech-language pathology, such as nursing and education, narrative inquiry has much more frequently been successfully and meaningfully used to explore the human phenomena relevant to those domains. In social work, another human service field, narrative inquiry has very rarely been applied and is in its early stages of development (Riesmann & Quinney, 2005). Generally in health care, however, narrative-based research and narrative techniques are being acknowledged as a means by which the humanness of living with illness or disability can be rightfully explored (Greenhalgh & Collard, 2003).

The role of qualitative research methods in general and narrative methods in particular can be clearly considered when we talk about the broad research paradigms in which research operates. Positivist and post-positivist paradigms hold in common that there is a reality or truth that can be sought or revealed, and that things can be known or unknown. Therefore, research methods including experimental methods, surveys, correlational studies, and rigorously defined qualitative studies might serve these purposes (Hatch, 2002). The products of these research endeavors include facts, theories, standards, and generalizations.

Of course, some would argue that even the most empirically-based quantitative approach is fraught with subjectivity. Researchers are humans, and thus their own internal conflicts, biases, and personalities no doubt affect which problems they choose to address in their research, and how they attack those problems and design and carry out experiments. "Too often the personal is represented in opposition to the objective, when the latter merely conceals the personal in pretentiousness," writes Okely (1996, p. 29).

A constructivist paradigm presumes that there are multiple realities that are co-constructed. Understanding comes from the interaction of the researcher and the participants creating meaning through dialogue and involvement. The products of this kind of paradigm and its associated research methods include case studies, narratives, and reflexive polyvocal texts (Hatch, 2002).

These paradigms and their associated research methodologies are different ways of knowing.

> Each of the ways of knowing, moreover, has operating principles of its own and its own criteria of well-formedness. They differ radically by their procedures for verification. A good story and a well-formed argument are different natural kinds. Both can be used as means for convincing another. Yet what they convince *of* is fundamentally different: arguments convince one of their truth, stories of their lifelikeness. The one verifies by eventual appeal to procedures for establishing formal and empirical proof. The other establishes not truth but verisimilitude. It has been claimed that the one is a refinement or an abstraction from the other. But this must be false or true only in the most unenlightening way (Bruner, 1986, p. 11).

Bruner (1986) argues that it is the intuitive, subjective narrative approach that generates hypotheses. More structured and formal qualitative approaches and quantitative methods have their use in testing hypotheses that may have emerged from qualitative and narrative explorations. The narrative approach generates stories that are embedded in the details of a particular context, whereas quantitative approaches aspire to generate broad conclusions and principles. Bruner continues:

> The imaginative application of the narrative mode leads instead to good stories, gripping drama, believable (though not necessarily "true") historical accounts. It deals in hopes or human-like intention and action and the vicissitudes and consequences that mark their course. It strives to put its timeless miracles into the particulars of experience, and to locate the experience in time and place. Joyce thought of the particularities of the story as epiphanies of the ordinary. The paradigmatic mode, by contrast, seeks to transcend the particular by higher and higher reaching for abstraction, and in the end disclaims in principle any explanatory value at all where the particular is concerned. There is a heartlessness to logic: one goes where one's premises and conclusions and observations take one . . . Paul Ricoeur argues that narrative is built upon concern for the human condition: stories reach sad or comic or absurd denouements, while theoretical arguments are simply conclusive or inconclusive" (Bruner, 1986, pp. 13–14).

The goal of lifelikeness in narrative approaches facilitates the links between narrative approaches and practical problems. "General normative principles are too abstract and crude to come to grips with practical problems" (Rosenwald & Ochberg, 1992, p. 278), but narrative techniques can grapple with highly specific and individualized issues.

Narrative is universal. There are three basic assumptions about the universalism of narrative (Hill, 2005). First, narrative is a link between a sequence of events and particular narrative sequences. Second, narrative is built from particular sets of clauses and structures. Third, narratives are a form of meaning-making, particularly between members of the same culture who share a particular understanding of the form and use of narratives. Narrative, and other aspects of talk and discourse, can reveal underlying cultural assumptions, beliefs, and perceptions (Quinn, 2005).

Stories are a common feature across cultures and across experiential boundaries; stories are experienced throughout the lifespan, in a variety of contexts. Stories can serve to cross a boundary in our field between science and practice, because stories can be used as a research tool that is strongly embedded in the details of a particular context, potentially illustrating how generalities or abstractions are played out in real contexts.

Purposes and Goals of Narrative Methodologies

Narrative methodologies share some basic characteristics with other research tools but, of course, offer their own distinctive contributions to certain research endeavors. Like every research tool, narrative methodologies are a form of persuasion. Narrative persuades us of its lifelikeness, whereas other quantitative efforts are aimed at persuading us of a truth. "Narrative, we suspect, is the most powerful mode of persuasion" (Brockmeir & Harre, 2001, p. 41). In almost every kind of communication context, from the informal to the formal, stories are used to illustrate and to persuade.

Like quantitative approaches, narrative methodologies have their own set of operating principles, and their own set of criteria for determining well-formedness. Quantitative approaches verify their resulting observations through procedures of reliability and replication. Verification occurs in narrative approaches, as well, and rests primarily on the determination of lifelikeness and verisimilitude. How well does the narrative technique represent the human phenomena that are its target?

Narrative approaches fill a distinctive niche within the range of research tools. Narrative inquiry, at its heart, is a way to delve into the human experience. Narrative approaches foreground individual characteristics, human intentions, and specific circumstances, revealing the particular (Clandinin & Connelly, 2000). In contrast, traditional quantitative methods strive to abstract generalities that can be applied and averaged across groups of individuals, transcending the particular. The contextual details in a narrative approach facilitate understanding human phenomena in relation to a particular cultural medium.

Narrative approaches provide a means to integrate human experience with contextualized details.

> Stories give room to doubt, anxiety, and hope as elements of concrete human interactions. Stories show intentions and

feelings as part of contextual and intersubjective ways of meaning making. They contain knowledge about practical solutions and show us patterns in practical life (Rosenwald & Ochberg, 1992, p. 277).

The role of narrative approaches in scientific inquiry can be summarized in two general points. First, narrative approaches are a rich soil in which to explore and generate hypotheses. Second, narrative approaches provide a technique for dialogue about topics otherwise difficult to address; these topics might include highly specific contexts, issues of individual variability, or explorations of human experience that is not quantifiable. Of course, narrative approaches have limits. These techniques do not generate the kind of weighty scientific evidence that is necessary for the creation of practice guidelines or standards, for example (Redman, 2005). But practice standards are generalized guidelines, and thus consistent with the goals of quantitative techniques.

Evidence-based practice is the search for general conclusions that are true; what treatment is best for whom under which circumstances. Thus, the search for evidence on which we can base general practice guidelines follows in a positivist paradigm and is associated with quantitative research methodologies and perhaps some tightly controlled qualitative research. Evidence-based practice can be described in a set of guidelines that steers the clinician to an appropriate integration of available scientific evidence with clinical experience. Evidence-based practice is predicated on the assumption that expert opinion alone is not sufficient for appropriate clinical decision making, and thus relies heavily on the weight of cumulative quantitative research. Typical outcomes of evidence-based practice are general standards and practice guidelines that are known to produce the most benefit for certain categories of patients. Thus evidence-based practice produces general conclusions specifically without regard for individual circumstances.

Narrative-based practice is the search for ways to acknowledge, learn from, and appropriately accommodate individual differences that come from cultural-linguistic backgrounds, personality, motivation, social support and context, attitudes and beliefs. Narrative-based practice fits within a constructivist paradigm and is tightly linked to case studies, narratives, interpretations, and reflexive writing including autoethnography.

Narrative-based approaches emphasize the individual's experience of illness or disability and firmly situate this experience within a specific set of cultural and environmental circumstances. Narrative-based approaches flesh out the bare bones of standards and guidelines derived from an evidence-based practice approach.

Clearly, these two approaches are most powerful when they can be used in a complementary and not antagonistic way. We do not say, when thinking about how to write a phrase on the page, "Is it better to use a period or a question mark?" The answer is dependent upon the purpose of the statement. Depending on our research assumptions, questions, and goals, different methodologies will produce the appropriate product.

Overview of Narrative Research Methods

There are many texts on qualitative research methods in general, and some techniques like interviewing and participant-observation are the topic of whole texts as well. The purpose in this single chapter, therefore, can only be to offer the reader a taste of some of the research tools that are characteristic of narrative approaches.

Some research procedures are common across the various narrative approaches. Two general categories of analysis are paradigmatic analysis and narrative analysis (Casey & Long, 2002, after Polkinghorne, 1995). In paradigmatic analysis, the researcher collects stories, and seeks to identify and describe common themes from across these stories. In this case, the researcher moves from stories to common elements with the goal to develop general knowledge about a collection of stories. In narrative analysis, the researcher collects descriptions of events and configures them into a plot or story, moving from elements to stories. One of the strengths of narrative analysis is preserving or identifying the individuality of stories.

In both cases, data collection includes the collection of descriptions or stories, and data analysis includes the analysis or synthesis of stories and their elements. Data collection often relies on observational techniques and interviews. Data analysis often relies on transcriptional approaches, conversational and discourse analysis, and triangulation to develop themes or identify important elements.

In some contexts—for example, in medical education—the more analytical narrative approach that tends to generate themes or common elements might be preferred because of an already existing rooting in the sciences (Bleakley, 2005). Analytical procedures tend to lose the detail and context that is a unique contribution of narrative approaches. Narrative synthesis can help to produce empathy and more holistic thinking (Bleakley, 2005).

Rhetorical analysis serves as the first example in this chapter; it is used as a tool to produce meta-narratives during a systematic review of the literature. Life narratives are another example described which relies on interviewing a particular sample of individuals and analyzing trends or themes across their life narratives. Finally, autoethnography is described as an example in which introspection and reflection produce a richly contextualized, detailed narrative that can address issues of individual experience.

Rhetorical Analysis

Greenhalgh et al. (2005) describe a rhetorically-based approach to conducting a systematic review of literature, in their case, a review of diffusion of innovation within health care. They describe the basic phases in their meta-narrative review. In the planning phase, a research team is formed, the outputs of the review are agreed upon, and a schedule is created for conducting the review and for research meetings. The search phase is characterized by three steps. Initially, researchers informally browse various literatures and search for potential publications through networking to increase the diversity and breadth of the literature that will ultimately be represented in the review. Seminal papers are then identified within the field. Finally, an electronic search aided by manual search is conducted for empirical papers. In the mapping phase, the key elements of the research paradigm, critical actors and researchers, and the prevailing language and imagery used by the scientists in each discipline are identified. Each primary study is then evaluated for its validity and relevance, and key results identified and summarized. At this point, the findings are synthesized by creating a narrative about how the topic has been studied and discussed in each discipline, including key actors and event sequences. Finally, the research team summarizes the overall messages of the research and distills recommendations for future research and for policy making.

In another example, Feldman, Skoldberg, Brown, and Horner (2004) describe a rhetorical analysis of stories told by city managers about successful and unsuccessful change in city management. In their technique, individuals within various levels of city management participate in unstructured interviews and the interviews are transcribed. Stories, defined as a sequence of events with a plot, are identified within the interviews, so that there may be many more stories within the data set than there are interviews. Stories were identified as a plot with a single theme that could be thought of as a response to the question, "And then what happened?"

After the successful identification of stories within the interviews, each story was analyzed on three levels. The first level was the identification of the basic point that the researcher thought the interviewee was making about the topic of the interview (change within the organization). This was also described as the story line. A brief summary or story line of the basic message of each story was created.

The second level of analysis involved the identification of oppositional themes. This second level of analysis was based on the assumption that most stories and their elements are told in an effort to differentiate the basic message from something that it is not. Although all stories did not seem to have opposition, most stories had single or multiple oppositions.

Third, the stories were analyzed from the point of view of a logical argument. The researchers attempted to create a logical syllogism from each story. A critical element in this analytic approach was the collaborative nature of the analysis; there were multiple researchers reviewing and analyzing the story lines, oppositions, and syllogisms. After this analysis was completed, thematic units were coded and data could be compared and sorted across stories and across different organizations.

Narrative inquiry is also being used as a means to investigate community health intervention programs. Stories are analyzed by their endpoints, characters, the actor/storyteller, the sequencing, and the tension created by the unfolding of the key events (Riley & Hawe, 2005).

Rhetorical analysis is a tool reliant on interviews or the reading of already published reports to generate a larger narrative. Typically, multiple researchers are used to seek agreement and a certain degree of reliability regarding the output of the analysis. Both of these processes are also present in the next research method, life narratives.

Life Narratives

Tedlock (2003) describes three forms of ethnographic genres that are relevant to a discussion of life narratives. The first is the *life history*, often generated from interviews but also from participant-observation in the field. The original premise of this form of work was that a single individual or family could represent a broader population or culture. A life history also provides the opportunity to describe an individual in a detailed context. A life history is defined as a retrospective account of an individual's life, in whole or in part, which overlaps with what is called the *biographical method* (Tierney, 2003). It has been suggested that a life history is produced when a researcher interprets a life story in a cultural context (Tierney, 2003). For some, the phrase *narrative case study* has been used to describe this genre. The narrative case study can be defined as "intensive examination of an individual unit," an individual, family, or other community (Brandell & Varkas, 2001, p. 294).

> ... the biographical method is similar to the lacy little country roads that allow the traveler to really discover the countryside, unlike the highways whose only merit is to bring one, more or less rapidly and safely, from one place to another while riding in the middle of nowhere (Voneche, 2001, p. 221).

A second important ethnographic genre is the *memoir*, in which an individual reflects about an important event or experience in the past. This form has generally been used to reflect on vivid events in a researcher's field experience. The memoir is linked conceptually to life narratives, but is a more direct ancestor of autoethnography, discussed in the next section.

A third ethnographic genre, the *narrative ethnography*, evolved from a blending of the life history and the memoir. In this form, researchers blend the account of a participant's life history with their own reactions or experiences. This blending of the participant's reflections with the researcher's reactions is the most common current representation of this style of work.

When researchers set out to produce narrative ethnographies of life histories, there are a number of means by which participants might be selected. First, the researcher may be involved in participant-observation, so that participants are those individuals with whom the researcher comes in contact. For example, if a researcher was participating in a support group, the participants might be those who happen to attend that particular support group. This could be considered an example of an opportunistic or convenience sample.

Another technique for selecting participants for interview-based methods is purposeful sampling. Criterion- or theory-driven samples are most familiar to those used to quantitative research. When interviewing is the data collection procedure of choice, Hatch (2002) describes the following possible strategies for selecting participants. First, one might select extreme or deviant case samples in which highly unusual examples of a characteristic is observed. In situations where contrasting viewpoints are of interest to the project, maximum variation samples involve individuals representing extreme, contrasting views on an issue. Typical case samples or homogenous samples represent what is considered to be usual in terms of a particular characteristic or phenomenon. Snowball or chain samples occur when one participant recommends another person who would be good to interview. Since qualitative approaches in general and narrative methods in particular are not attempting to test a hypothesis or select a sample that is representative of a population, purposeful sampling can accomplish the goal of including participants who share a particular trait or experience that is of interest to the researcher.

Data are collected, for life narratives, through interviews (Mishler, 1986). Hatch (2002) describes three kinds of interviews. The first kind is the formal interview. Formal interviews are also known as *structured interviews*. In these interviews, the researcher typically sets a time limit for the interview and approaches the interview with a set of guiding questions. Standardized interviews are a special subtype of formal interviews. In this interview type, researchers ask the same set of questions, in the same order, with the same wording, to each participant. Standardized interviews are considered a form of qualitative research because they generate data that are not in the form of closed-class response sets, and provide participants with open-ended opportunities to disclose information. In all forms of formal interviews, both participants and researchers recognize that they have entered into the conversation or interview with the purpose to generate data.

The informal interview is defined as unstructured conversations that occur within the research context. Informal interviews must comply with appropriate consent procedures, to be sure; but because of their informal style, a data-driven purpose is less evident. Both researcher and participant may more freely participate in an informal interview style.

Semi-structured interviews allow the researcher to act outside an originally planned question script. In this case, the researcher often probes for additional information or follows up on topics initiated by the participant that are outside the questions set before the interview. *In-depth interviews* are generally included in this category, because a set of general questions guides the interviewer initially, but the researcher is free to pursue more information on topics or events that are brought up by the participant.

Interviews for life narratives or narrative ethnographies can take a number of forms, but generally in-depth interviewing techniques are employed when the topic of interest is the life story. The three-interview series is one example of a procedure associated with in-depth interviewing (Seidman, 2006). In the first interview, the participant is asked how he or she came to do or be involved in what is of interest to the researcher; to put the characteristic or activity of interest in the broader context of the life story. The focus of the second interview is to describe in detail the topic of interest to the study. The purpose here is to reconstruct the details, however mundane, of the activities of interest. In the third interview, the participant is asked to reflect on the meaning of the topic of interest. The researcher should focus on the sense or meaning that the participant has made of the activities or events described in the previous two interviews.

The reader is no doubt reminded here of the three-session Pennebaker therapeutic writing paradigm, in which participants are asked to write about an emotional event over the course of three to five sessions. The typical course of the therapeutic writing includes a basic reporting of events, inclusion of additional details, and finally reflection on the meaning of the events and how the associated emotions have affected the construction of their subsequent life. In research as in therapeutic activities, repetition of the story provides an opportunity for processing and meaning-making.

It also becomes clear, then, why some researchers have observed that asking individuals to participate in a series of interviews about a critical life event has been reported by the participants as positive and, for some, therapeutic (Grinyer, 2004; Rosenwald, 1996).

An example of in-depth interviewing is provided by Sells, Topor, and Davidson (2004). Two individuals recovering from mental illness were interviewed and the transcripts were analyzed by five investigators. The researchers conducted independent readings of the transcripts, identified important themes, temporally ordered those themes, and developed consensus regarding their analyses. The process yielded a fruitful way to understand issues of recovery in the details of an individual's life.

Another example of a research tool that has been applied in the health domain is Video Intervention/Prevention Assessment (VIA) (Rich & Patashnick, 2002). This is a software package that accommodates videotaped illness narratives and video diaries of those living with and managing chronic illnesses. These techniques allow multiple researchers to tag or log analyses on videotaped journals of patients, and can therefore allow participants the freedom of expression available in a video diary format while offering data management power.

Life narratives, and in particular narrative ethnographies that incorporate the participant's story and the researcher's reactions to it, are frequently used to help researchers understand the extent of influence of an experience on subsequent life events and life meaning. Participant selection techniques and interview procedures may vary across studies or purposes. But in every case the researcher is an acknowledged presence in the study; an individual is telling his or her life story to that particular researcher in the particular place and time for some understood reason.

Autoethnography

Autoethnography is a relatively new development within the range of narrative ethnographic tools. The *auto* in autoethnography refers to the use of the self as a source within a narrative form that portrays some aspect of lived experience. Autoethnography is "a form of self-narrative that places the self in a social context" (Reed-Danahay, 1997, p. 6).

Autoethnography shares characteristics of autobiography and ethnographic narrative. The writer uses introspective techniques (Ellis, 1991) to reflect on an event or experience, and attempts to integrate the emotions experienced at the time of the event with the reflections that have evolved over the passage of time since the event. Thus, autoethnography is more than just a retelling of life events like an autobiography. Autoethnography includes an evocative and perhaps analytical reflection on the event, characteristic of ethnographic narratives.

In order to sort this out a bit more clearly, let's consider some definitions. Here is a working definition of autobiography:

> A narrator, in the here and now, takes upon himself or herself the task of describing the progress of a protagonist in the there and then, one who happens to share his name. He must by convention bring that protagonist from the past into the present in such a way that the protagonist and the narrator eventually become one person with a shared consciousness (Bruner, 2001, p. 27).

The ethnographic portion of autoethnography is the incorporation of the researcher's perspective, consciously, in the form and/or content of the text. One of the earliest reports of incorporating the researcher's view into a report of communication disorder is "A Glimpse into an Aphasic's World," by Eleanor T. Albertson, published in the *American Journal of Occupational Therapy* in 1947. She describes a moment when she was first introduced to a patient with aphasia; as her director said, "The patient has difficulty in expressing himself." She reports that she felt like laughing because it struck her as a "common enough difficulty." She reports that during the time that she got to know this particular patient, she came to learn about aphasia. In addition to outlining tasks and activities that the staff at her hospital designed during World War II to help patients with aphasia, she suggests: "Probably the greatest help a therapist can give to an aphasic is the desire to accept himself for the present as he is, while he continues to work for maximum improvement." And she wisely concludes: "For I rather imagine it's important that we don't *wait* to become what we should like to be, but do our *living* now, letting it be a growing and a very satisfying and exciting thing" (p. 364). This writing is a very clear example of specifically and consciously including the observer's viewpoint in the text. This same perspective is integrated in an ethnographic fashion with one's own experiences in an autoethnography.

There are many possible purposes of autoethnography. Not each autoethnographic narrative strives to accomplish each of these, but the body of autoethnographic work that now exists probably includes these as goals (see Ellis, 2004, an entire textbook devoted to autoethnography). Self-knowledge may be a goal of autoethnography, not just for the writer but for those readers who interact with the text and recognize some of themselves within it. Auto-ethnographies can be used to tell a story, illustrate a concept, or reflect on a state or culture. Autoethnography can focus attention on the mundane—what Joyce referred to as "epiphanies of the ordinary." There is an "Aha!" experience for the writer and/or the reader. Perhaps "Aha! I never thought of it that way," or "Aha! Now I have an idea what that must be like," or "Aha! I've never come so close to imaging the horror/wonder of that."

Autoethnographies are written in a self-reflective, evocative mode, and this requires a few procedures (Ellis, 1997). First, there is generally some temporal distance between the lived event and the writing of the autoethnography. The amount of time that passes between the two things is individual-specific. But there is clearly a difference between writing that occurs during an experience (like journal writing during a crisis) and the kind of writing that occurs after sufficient time has passed to allow both for separation and reflection along with the courage to relive the event through evocative writing.

Some have argued that it is indeed the passage of time that facilitates the creation of narrative out of life events, the perception of sequence from what may have been coincidental.

> ... autobiographical narrative tends to lose an essential dimension of human life: chance. "Lived time" appears to be a sort of direct linkage between two well-defined moments in time. In this manner, the uncertainty and arbitrariness of life seems to be absorbed, and the plurality of options, realized or not, which is so characteristic of human agency is inevitably reduced to a simple chain of events. . . . Molded in a tight narrative fabric, the story makes the life as a unified whole . . . (Freeman, 2001, p. 253).

Is there a difference between journalism, fiction, and something in between? Current soldiers stationed in Iraq and Afghanistan are writing blogs, and at least one blog writer has contracted to publish the first "blook," or book coming from an ongoing blog. Colby Buzzell wrote *My War: Killing Time in Iraq,* published in October 2005. One criticism of this kind of publication is that it lacks a time lag between the experience and the writing, so that no analysis or reflection can be incorporated into the writing. Nathaniel Fick, another soldier-author whose book *One Bullet Away: The Making of a Marine Officer* was also published in October 2005, also wrote his stories down as soon as he returned from a tour of duty in Iraq. He says, "A book with 20, 30 years reflection is a different book from mine. Not that either one is better or worse—just a different book. I thought that if I had waited, I would have lost some of the emotional immediacy" ("Combat Inspires Soldiers to Pick Up a Pen," *Miami Herald*, November 14, 2005).

In contrast, stories that have the benefit of several years of reflection are "distilled," in the way that water is distilled. The elements have evaporated and rough spots or irrelevant minerals separated, and the pure hydrogen-oxygen combination remains.

Another important aspect of autoethnography is that these narratives are written with the goal to evoke similar experiences in the readers, and thus literary techniques are used to accomplish this.

> The delight we experience when we allow ourselves to respond to a fairy tale, the enchantment we feel comes not from the psychological meaning of a tale (although this contributes to it) but from its literary qualities—the tale itself as a work of art. The fairy tale could not have its psychological impact on the child were it not first and foremost a work of art (Bettelheim, 1976, p. 12).

Literary techniques are used freely to target literary truth or the reproduction of lifelikeness.

Literary truth implies that the text gets at the real meaning or experience that is being communicated. This can be differentiated from historical truth, in which the sequence of facts such as chronology and objective events is retold in the form of technical writing. In autoethnography, the goal is literary truth so that a variety of art forms—including plays, poetry, and a variety of tools within prose—are employed by the researcher to capture and convey lived experience.

But even historical truth, conveyed in an evocative manner, has as its goal the recreation of a particular event. "The work of the historian consists of the re-experiencing of a transmitted event into which he or she has projected him- or herself and that he or she has re-created and thus consciously relived" (Laub, 2006, p. 256). Historical truth or factual accuracy can be successfully combined with literary truth to evoke the full sense of an experience.

Stories must be written in a form that brings art and reason or information to the targeted audience. Without the art of the story, only the intellect is appealed to; the art appeals to the emotional aspect of the reader. A fairy tale would not achieve the goal of addressing both emotive and intellectual issues for the adult clinician—but a true story with literary or fictionalized aspects meets this need, like the fairy tale meets the need of the young child.

Autoethnography is judged based on its ability to achieve the goal of lifelikeness.

Effective autoethnography should be evocative and self-reflexive, creating an authentic dialogue between the writer and the reader (Behar, 1997; Ellis, 1997; Sparkes, 2000; Spry, 2001). Autoethnography can be judged on its evocativeness, because its usefulness in a professional domain should be based on whether readers are led to a similar experience as the writer through a reading of the narrative (Ellis, 1995; Sparkes, 2000).

Ethical Considerations in Narrative Research

Research should do no harm. This is the ethical kernel that guides us as we conduct all of our professional practices. In every case, the risks for potential harm have to be weighed against the potential for benefit. The risk-benefit ratio for any given research or practice should be conceptualized as a continuum; at some point a higher risk with a lower potential for benefit is no longer "worth it."

But in a qualitative research paradigm and in narrative methods in particular, there are risks for harm that are sometimes difficult to identify. What may seem like a relatively innocuous activity could produce harmful effects to the psyche of a participant, or negatively influence the social circle in which the participant lives.

These potentials for harm can sometimes be anticipated but at other times are very difficult to anticipate.

For example, Barnard (2005) describes the potential for harm in a narrative ethnographic study in which drug addicted mothers were interviewed about their child care practices in an effort to explore the effects of drug use on child-rearing. Some of the children of these mothers were also interviewed about their experiences. Barnard (2005) writes about the potential for harm that participation in the interview could cause, and how the interviewers at times avoided probing some topics further because of the researcher's perspective that it might be inappropriate or personally wrong. Questions and probes about some experiences could cause the participants to confront issues that were previously avoided mentally and psychologically, and without appropriate judgment about when to stop, potential psychological harm on sensitive topics could be caused. In this particular research context, interview probes that were perceived as problematic by the researchers were questions that asked the participants to elaborate on events that were seemingly sources of guilt and pain regarding neglect of their children because of drug use. The researchers perceived an ethical issue that was not anticipated when they began the study regarding how to conduct these unstructured interviews and what questions to ask.

An alternative view is offered by a follow-up study of parents of young adults with cancer who had contributed narrative accounts to a research project (Grinyer, 2004). In the follow-up, parents reflected that they had found their research participation positive and that the writing of narratives was therapeutic. In addition, the parents indicated that they experienced less social isolation as a result of participating in the project. The parents did express, however, that there was a high level of emotional demand caused by remembering, reflecting on, and revealing painful memories for the purpose of research. This report seemed to suggest that, at least in some cases, participants perceive that good came out of what was a somewhat difficult activity to complete (see also Rosenwald, 1996).

The extent and depth of the emotions expressed in an in-depth interview may not have been anticipated either by the participant or by the researcher, and can therefore become a source of potential ethical concern (Goodman, 2001). Professional boundaries may become blurred particularly if the interview is of a conversational or informal nature. Therapeutic interventions must be avoided in the researcher-participant relationship, and participants referred for appropriate follow-up services if necessary (Goodman, 2001).

Because ethnographic research relies on the researcher as the primary data collection instrument and is based on a personal interaction between the researcher and the participant, special ethical considerations ensue. Roper and Shapira (2000) discuss three areas of concern for ethical practice in ethnographic research. Biases of the researchers must be identified. This can be done through awareness and self-monitoring, and by including the emotional reactions of the researcher into the research report in one of a variety of ways. In participant research, the researcher may play the role of an outsider but gradually over time may develop an insider perspective. The representation of the insider perspective is an important and critical aspect of ethnographic research. When researchers have carefully tracked their own reactions, particularly as they progress from an outsider role to an insider, potential biases can be acknowledged and discussed.

Informed consent is another area in which special ethical considerations sometimes occur that are different from those in typical quantitative research methods. In a typical quantitative experiment, participants consent and then fairly quickly participate in a structured activity that is often relatively short in duration and participation time. Qualitative methods and narrative approaches in particular observe participants over lengthy periods of time during which they are usually revealing information of a personal nature. Informed consent, then, must be an *ongoing* process in ethnographic research rather than a single-time event. Participants initially consent to being interviewed or observed, depending on the nature of the study. The stories that are generated, however, may be revealing of intimate details of individuals' lives. Before these data are published or disseminated in any way, it is important for the researcher to clarify with the participants the nature of the dissemination and whether the participants continue to consent to a sharing of the information in the form that the researcher is proposing.

The respect and maintenance of confidentiality can be a tricky issue in ethnography, since by definition ethnographic narratives include a high degree of contextualized detail, and this detail alone may be sufficient to suggest a participant's identity in a way that breaches agreements of confidentiality. The use of pseudonyms and the changing of important participant characteristics does not always protect the participant from undesired identification, since details about location, timeline of events, and many other contexts could lead readers to successfully guess about the participant.

There are additional ways, beyond the use of pseudonyms, which can aid the researcher in ensuring that participants are not unintentionally harmed by a breach of confidentiality. One classic example in ethnography is the use of composite characters or fictionalized versions of experiences as a way to completely mask the details of participants. These techniques preserve the literary truth of the researcher's experiences but change the historical truth in ways that would not allow readers to identify a particular individual in the resulting narrative. Angrosino (1998) used this technique when he wrote about his participant-observer experiences volunteering in a group home for people with developmental disabilities. Because he felt that writing about the characteristics of any of the clients in the group home would endanger privacy, he wrote his ethnography using composite characters and fictionalized versions of bits and pieces of clients that he had known, while still communicating his experiences.

Alternatively, the participants might choose to be directly involved in the writing process. Another technique that some researchers have used is to ask participants to review the draft of the proposed narrative to be disseminated, and to systematically provide the participants with an opportunity to approve or disapprove particular details or aspects of the narrative that are suggestive of their identity or are revealing of them in some other way. Ethnographers who use this technique often write letters to the participants and ask them to respond in writing, or hold additional conversations with the participants to get their feedback on the narrative draft. On two occasions when I have used this approach, both participants ended by insisting that their real name be used in the publication. Clearly, in other instances researchers have experienced the opposite reaction, in which participants have rescinded their consent or asked that particular details be changed to avoid identification.

In any case, though, the primary principle is to respect the confidentiality of the participants. When doing ethnographic research, we must be cognizant that our participants may not fully appreciate the potential ramifications of publishing data from their stories. The typical informational item on an informed consent form is generally vague and might refer to scientific publications. And although we are assuming that our participants might not be affected by a publication in one of our scientific journals, we really don't know who among their family, friends, or acquaintances might come across such a publication. It's a little like chatting about clients in a coffee house—you never know who is sitting behind you and whether they might know that client, even if you don't use the name. The best practice, then, is to confer with participants as much as is practicable in an ongoing process, and to use our finest-tuned ethical judgments when dealing with the kind of data and observations that come from narrative modes of research.

STUDY/DISCUSSION QUESTIONS AND ACTIVITIES

1. Have you ever experienced the retelling of a story that involved you but conveyed what you felt was an unflattering view? Reflect on and discuss your experience.
2. Discuss the possible applications of rhetorical analysis, life narratives, or autoethnography to the exploration of particular research areas in speech-language pathology.
3. What reactions do you have to the basic tenets or assumptions associated with qualitative research in general and narrative research in particular? Be honest about your own biases or reactions and discuss them.

5

Illness and Disability Narratives

OVERVIEW

One particular type of narrative, illness narrative, is particularly relevant to the consideration of narrative in the lives of clients with communication disorder. Illness and disability narratives have been studied in medical anthropology, communication, and health science. Typical forms of these narratives are described. Illness narratives seem to produce curative effects for those who tell them and also reveal the experience of developing coping strategies and making meaning from illness or disability.

LEARNING OBJECTIVES

At the end of this chapter, the reader will be able to:

1. Define illness narrative.

2. List and describe three categories of illness narrative, according to Frank (1995).

3. Discuss at least three aspects of living with illness or disability that can be revealed through illness/disability narratives.

Illness Narratives

Narratives are the way we make sense of the sequence of events in our lives, how we enfold ourselves in our cultural backgrounds while asserting our individuality, and relate to others by projecting ourselves in the role they play. A traumatic event like illness or disability requires its own set of meaning-making and coping efforts. Meta-narratives exist in the dominant medical culture and in our own cultural backgrounds that offer a formula for talking about and dealing with illness and disability. Because the onset of illness or disability is often self-defining, narratives of illness are often vivid accounts that reflect the individual grappling with issues within a specific cultural context. Illness narratives reveal our culture's view of living with illness or disability and each individual's reaction to this set of circumstances. Because illness and disability are events that can befall anyone without warning, they are of interest to everyone. Even healthy people are curious about what it is like when illness occurs.

Illness narratives, like all narratives, are socially constructed. The context of the telling—who it is told to, why, when, and where—contributes to the characteristics of the narrative. The illness narrative cannot be divorced from the life story of the individual (Beck, 2005).

Illness narratives are told from one person to another in intimate moments, told in support groups, written and published, or told through other media like film and television. Much of the public's medical knowledge comes from television programs, including documentaries, soap operas, and other serials, and it is through these avenues that most of the public comes in contact with illness narratives. Some media presentations are more credible or are judged by the public as more valuable than others (Davin, 2003). It seems that some illness narratives as portrayed in certain media, such as some soap operas, are viewed as less lifelike and contain less narrative truth than others.

In the sections that follow, the definition, forms, and categories of illness narratives will be reviewed. Examples of the purposes and meanings of illness narratives will be described, and the potential role of these narratives in speech-language pathology will be suggested.

Definition of Illness Narratives

An illness narrative is the story a person tells about how he became ill, what first made him think something was wrong, what help was sought, how doctors and other health professionals responded, and what treatment was recommended and pursued. An important part of an illness narrative is the individual's emotional reactions, intentions, motivations, and inner experiences during diagnosis and treatment. A listener wants to know how the person feels now, what has the illness meant to him, whether it has changed his life, and if so, in what ways. It is the story of personal experience and meaning that differentiate an illness narrative from a typical case presentation in a traditional medical style.

A life narrative is often elicited in an unstructured interview format, and the same is true for an illness narrative. Like other stories of traumatic events, illness narratives come in various forms and evolve depending on how much time has passed in relation to the events being retold, in what context the story is being told, and how many times the story has been retold.

The illness narrative is a particular genre of story, because it forms a bridge between the ideal life and real circumstances (Skultans, 1998; Riessman, 1993). These circumstances are founded within the cultural context, and illness narratives can inform us about others' perceptions of health, illness, and coping within their society.

For example, Skultans (1998; 1997a; 1997b) shows how individual illness narratives of Latvian women are embedded in societal perceptions of the shortcomings of the Soviet regime in post-war Latvia. Each individual's narrative is a telling of particular circumstances, but it often refers back to social issues or problems including inadequately diagnosed illnesses or poor treatment decisions.

Narratives generated from interviews of Hong Kong Chinese men and women reveal the mix of Western and Eastern philosophies that influence their conception of health and medical care (Chan, Cheung, Mok, Cheung, & Tong, 2006). The question, "What is it like to be healthy?" and related questions were posed in interviews and the narrative responses analyzed for themes. It appeared from the sample of participants in this study that some participants were viewing issues of health from a mix of Chinese and Western perspectives. The narratives revealed the links between their understandings of health and their cultural viewpoints, and the results suggested directions for future health education and promotion activities. For example, the respondents talked about health in the context of the family and implications for health and illness in relation to family members. Thus, health education activities that emphasize the family might be a successful potential avenue to pursue.

Besides a broader view of culture, the more immediate cultural context of a relationship also serves as a medium in which health and illness narratives are constructed. Couples in long-term relationships co-construct joint illness narratives in relation to the illness or disability of one spouse. These narratives are created within the context of the relationship culture. In one study, five couple styles emerged: the sympathetic couple, the independent couple, the rejecting couple, the nonreciprocal couple, and the mixed couple (Walker & Dickson, 2004). The way in which a couple jointly tells the story of an experienced illness reveals how the couple has coped with the illness.

Illness provides an opportunity to explore individual and cultural aspects of coping with a trauma that is equally possible to everyone. It is not a narrative that is exclusively for soldiers, women who have given birth, firefighters, or some other group identified by a shared characteristic. Every human has become ill, or is going to become ill, or has someone close to him who has been ill.

Types of Illness Narratives

Illness narratives occur in all possible narrative forms, of course; narratives are told orally, written in journals, published as books and articles, told in film and television media, and shared on the Internet on personal Web pages, blogs, and *blooks* (blogs published in the form of books). Regardless of the format of the illness narrative, the story may take a fairly predictable overall course. These general categories of illness narratives derive from cultural viewpoints and reflect cultural standards and expectations about being ill or disabled.

More than 10 years ago, the work of Arthur Frank brought illness experiences and illness narratives to the attention of sociologists and others interested in what the experience of illness reveals to us about our own culture and everyday experience. He claims that his first book (Frank, 1991) was not intended to be a scientific approach to illness but rather a personal reflection of his own experiences (Frank, 2004). His later work (for example, Frank, 1995) brought qualitative methods of inquiry to bear on the human phenomenon of being ill.

Frank (1995) proposed three general categories of illness narratives. Quest narratives, the most frequently occurring and perhaps most acceptable type of illness narrative in Western culture, are those in which the person perceives the illness or disability as a journey, in which some kind of meaning is sought. In her published narrative about living with stroke and aphasia, Perez (2001) illustrates the quest narrative in her description of her experience as a journey.

> My own journey to "stroke-land" was different from any journey I'd taken before, but it was worth all the effort because I learned to laugh at myself and to trust myself. Before the stroke, I wouldn't have been able to see a brain attack as an opportunity for growth, but it gave me the chance to delve deep inside myself and find that I was tougher than I thought possible (p. 221).

Restitution narratives are those that focus on the details of the medical process and treatment, and the focus is returning to the previous state of health. These stories are full of treatment details. The restitution narrative follows three basic segments: health lost, a cure found, and health restored. Such a narrative may occur most frequently in the early stages of long or chronic illness or disability. In the case of a terminal illness such as cancer, clinging to a restitution narrative may postpone decisions about hospice care and hinder participation in life-ending activities (Myers, 2002). The restitution narrative prolongs hope in a cure rather than emphasizing the creation of meaning at the end of life and hope for quality at end of life. The quest narrative may provide a more hopeful and realistic theme for managing quality of life in terminal illness.

Chaos narratives reflect the loss of control and disruption of life that come about as a result of illness or disability. One of the most potent metaphors conveying a sense of chaos was written by Robert McCrum, who experienced stroke and speech disorder, in his book, *My Year Off* (1999).

> . . . I say that sometimes I feel like the pilot of an aeroplane who on looking over his shoulder in the cockpit sees his tail-plane and the end of his fuselage suddenly blown away, but who finds, amazingly, that although his plane has gone into a 'graveyard spin', somehow it has not crashed. Today, I feel like a pilot who is nursing his crippled craft to a safe landing somewhere unfamiliar, but close at hand (McCrum, 1999, p. 215).

Chaos narratives occur infrequently, probably because they are not condoned socially and culturally as are quest and restitution narratives.

These broad categories of illness narratives might be produced by the same individual at different times during the course of illness or adjusting to disability. Different types of illness narratives might be produced in relation to the person one is talking with or other contextual variables. And of course, the production of these different categories of illness narrative might be related to the individual's personality, family background, and cultural perspective.

Recently, the narratives of adults living with aphasia after stroke that had been published on Internet Web sites were analyzed and responded to by a group of aphasia researchers and their co-researchers, a group of people living with aphasia (Moss, Byng, Parr, & Petheram, 2004). The people with aphasia who evaluated stories of living with aphasia on various Web sites indicated a preference for those stories that were motivating and positive, primarily quest narratives. These positive narratives showed how individuals had made meaning in their lives after the onset of aphasia. When the group of co-researchers made their own stories for possible publication on the Internet, some of them produced restitution narratives, a form of narrative that had been criticized by the group when they had considered others' narratives.

This suggests an interesting difference between social or cultural preference and individual experience. As a group, the quest narrative was preferred, and this is consistent with Frank's (1995) observation that the quest narrative is the most culturally consistent form of illness narrative among Western cultures. But although the group of co-researchers, all individuals living with aphasia, had reviewed different styles and forms of personal narratives, their own stories did not necessarily conform to what they found most encouraging or comforting to read or listen to. Thus the telling of an illness narrative, in this case the story of living with a communication disorder, seems to be an avenue for processing one's individual circumstances, and more than likely reveals stages of coping and adaptation to the illness. We are uncomfortable listening to stories that highlight what we might consider to be unrealistic expectations or lack of adjustment, even though these might be the current state of our own internal affairs.

Three characteristics of narratives are perhaps interesting ways to consider different types of illness narratives (Weingarten & Weingarten Worthen, 1999). Narrative coherence is the congruent interrelationships between the plot, characters, and themes within the story. Weingarten and Weingarten Worthen's (1999) interwoven story is about a mother experiencing breast cancer when her daughter was age 9 years. The daughter had been diagnosed with Beckwith-Wiedeman syndrome, a rare syndrome that is little known even in the medical establishment. They observe how the mother's breast cancer story was highly coherent, because the plot sequence is relatively well fixed and all the characters (health professionals, patient, and patient's family) are experiencing emotions against a shared backdrop of this sequence of events. Incoherence was experienced in terms of the daughter's story, because the sequence of events for Beckwith-Wiedeman syndrome is unknown and unfamiliar to all the characters in the story.

A second feature of narratives is narrative closure, and this element can also vary across different types of illness narratives. Narrative closure refers to the singularity of the story's interpretation, and how resistant the story is to alternative interpretations. Closure comes from completeness and cultural resonance. So, in the case of a breast cancer narrative, most individuals are likely to have a relatively complete understanding of the typical story; they know, generally, what cancer is and how it is treated. The typical breast cancer story, too, is one of triumph or attempt to triumph over illness and adversity, and this quest narrative form is consistent with cultural expectations. In contrast, little if anything was known about the daughter's Beckwith-Wiedeman syndrome, and so individuals who played roles in the story filled in gaps of understanding and knowledge in various ways. Not understanding the meaning of some symptoms of the syndrome, individuals tended to associate the symptoms with things that they thought they knew about. Weingarten and Weingarten Worthen (1999) give the example here of the large tongue that is typically associated with the syndrome. Many individuals associated larger tongues with mental retardation, although mental retardation is not associated with this particular syndrome. Thus the lack of narrative completeness meant that there were various possible interpretations of pieces of the story that were not always beneficial.

Many communication disorders are little understood or even misunderstood by many. These gaps in knowledge are filled in, perhaps in nonproductive ways. Individuals living with communication disorders then experience the results of this lack of information—being misidentified as retarded, drunk, or otherwise "not right." Furthermore, many communication disabilities improve slowly and do not ever completely "go away." So the story is not as culturally appealing in the West as the story of the triumphant breast cancer survivor who fought through treatment and survived to a critical time point. When we consider how to educate the public about communication disorders, perhaps we should take into account the kind of story that is most likely to be successfully waved as a banner. Although that story is not everyone's story, the first step is to get a representative story out to the public that would help to educate them about the basics of any particular communication disorder.

The third aspect of narrative that is important to illness narratives is narrative interdependence. Interdependence is how stories of interacting individuals interrelate. Narratives of family members dealing with illness or disability in a single member may show various degrees of interdependence, and this might reveal something about the family's culture as well as each individual's experience.

Purposes and Meanings of Illness Narratives

Illness narratives are pervasive—everyone tells the story of his illness or disability. So obviously, telling these stories must hold purposes or meanings to the tellers. The literature on illness narratives suggests that telling the story of one's illness produces important benefits. There are also benefits to those—clinicians and researchers—who listen to illness narratives. In the next two sections these two broad interpretations of illness narratives are described.

Curative Effects of Illness Narratives

Illness narratives are themselves a form of healing, and can produce psychological and psychosocial benefits, just in their telling. Telling the story of one's illness or disability can help one to formulate or reformulate the trajectory of one's life. It can reduce social isolation; even listening to others' stories about their experiences with the same or similar health challenges can have healing effects. Finally, formulating the story of one's illness can play a role in changing the role of the patient from a passive recipient of care to an active part of the health care process.

Illness is a potential biographical disruption because it is, for most people, unexpected and unplanned; it is not included in the outline of the future chapters of one's life. (I suppose it could be said, then, that hypochondriacs have created a personal story that is centered on being ill. In that case, a bout of health might be a disruption in their particular biographical flow.) We have already made mention of the fact that disruption of one's life trajectory may be dependent on age and life development issues. The example was previously given of older adults who experience stroke, and the observation that stroke was not as much of a disruption to their life narrative as might be expected (Faircloth, Boylstein, Young, & Gubrium, 2004). This is quite different, however, for young people.

Narratives of young men and women experiencing remission from serious illness reveal that these stories are a social mechanism by which the young person constructs or reconstructs identity after facing serious illness and potential early death (Drew, 2003). Young people who are survivors combine fear and hope in considering potential future life courses and events, as they weave a story of their current circumstances and extrapolate to the future. Illness narratives of young survivors of serious illness are particularly characterized by issues of reconstructing the self and reconceptualizing the future. To a certain extent, young people are generally more involved in creating their own identities, whether they have been ill or not. Narratives both produce the opportunity for young adults to construct views of their own identities and also reveal how their illness experiences affect their identity construction and life planning.

In the case of older adults, their identity rests on decades of self-perceptions and a long history of events. Thus it is conceivable that an illness, no matter how disabling or traumatic, might not substantially change the story they tell about their whole life or their identity. But it does seem that older adults would need to renegotiate their current and future social roles.

In speech-language pathology, Shadden (2005) argues that identity renegotiation is essential in the case of living with aphasia after stroke and Sacks (2005) eloquently describes this problem. It would not surprise me at all if communication disorders, perhaps generally, were more acutely interwoven with identity renegotiation than other forms of disability. Our voice, speech, and language become projections of ourselves, like our name. When some aspect of our communication ability is affected, our ability to portray ourselves to the world in the way we have become accustomed to is changed, and thus this acutely affects the social construction of our identity. Similarly, for those whose communication disorder has existed from an early age, the communication disorder is part of the social fabric in which the child is developing. The explicit or implied stories that the child hears about his or her communication disability will become part of the story that he tells himself, and becomes part of his identity. Listening to the stories of children who are growing up with ongoing communication disabilities could potentially have positive benefits for the children, and aid them in negotiating their own identity and life course construction. It would also be revealing to speech-language pathologists and all those who are interested in facilitating both the communication and overall psychological development of children with communication disabilities. This is an area that deserves greater research attention in our field.

Telling the story of one's illness or disability can reduce social isolation because telling the story is of itself a social constructivist process. Each time the story is told, it is told to some particular audience, with some general intent and context; even if the narrative is being formed in a journal, there is an imagined audience and context. This benefit of telling one's illness narrative may at least partially explain why individuals living with illness or disability retell their story. By telling the story, they may come upon those who have similar experiences or who are at least sympathetic to their circumstances, and this decreases the feeling of being on one's own in an unfamiliar country.

My husband experienced a sudden and relatively serious bout of labyrinthitis, an inner ear infection that essentially caused him to feel severely seasick in his home. Before he came down with the infection, we had only read about the illness in audiology textbooks. But after he became ill and recovered over a period of several weeks, the telling of the story of how he became ill and what symptoms he experienced to our neighbors and friends resulted in a surprising number of people who said they had had labyrinthitis, too! We had no idea that any of these people had experienced the same illness, but as we repeated the story, we were surprised at how many times the response was, "Oh yeah, my wife had that, too!" Repeating the story of his labyrinthitis made us feel that many people in our social circle understood the recovery process and were sympathetic to our circumstances.

Even listening to others' stories has its own healing effect (Frank, 1995). Continuing with the case of my husband, the telling of his illness narrative often elicited a reciprocal telling of the other person's narrative. Listening to the details of their stories helped us to understand the possible range of symptoms and severity levels that could be experienced, and helped us to gauge where within that range my husband's illness fit. According to the Desiderata, one should never compare oneself to others, "for there will always be those who are greater and lesser than yourself." But when one is experiencing a relatively uncommon illness or disability—as are all of the communication disorders—listening to the stories of others helps us to gain a better appreciation of ourselves and how our disability could be worse or better. Honestly, though, even when we are experiencing the common cold, we want to hear the stories of others who have recently had the latest bug and consider how our 5 days of nose-blowing compares.

Finally, telling the story of one's illness can help one to remain active in the health care process. In other words, the telling of the story provides a sense of agency and of ownership of the process. It prevents the situation in which others—perhaps doctors, speech-language pathologists, or other health care professionals—are creating a story for you.

When we give our clients an opportunity to tell us about themselves, about their communication, and about what is troubling them, we are asking them to tell us the story of their illness or disability. Sometimes because of policy or logistical constraints, we have much less time for allowing our clients to tell their own illness story than we would like. But the chance to produce a communication disability narrative may produce its own positive results, in creating a positive social connection and providing an opportunity to reformulate the story of one's life and the story of adapting to the communication disability.

Revelatory Aspects of Illness Narratives

Illness narratives also show others how illness relates to culture and the individual's experience, and how individuals perceive these themes together. Illness narratives can reveal the individual's knowledge about an illness or disability, and show how the illness is understood or misunderstood. As the person explains his own illness, we come to see how he understands the illness. Narratives also have the potential to share the details of coping with a disability. Thus illness narratives can inform those of us who are not experiencing a particular illness or disability (yet) about the experience, and this in turn can have an impact on how we offer services, provide health education, or design interventions.

When a person tells the story of his own illness or disability, the story often includes a segment about how the illness started and what the perceived causes were or must have been. When the cause is unclear, the story often includes a portion about all the reasons why that particular illness should not have occurred to that person, and an indication of how puzzling or mysterious it is to have had it occur. Illness narratives often focus on explaining the onset of illness or disability.

When children are born with developmental disabilities, or congenital anomalies such as cleft palate, a major focus of attention particularly on the part of parents' narratives is why this has occurred to their child. Science is making progress on describing how all of these disabilities occur from a biological point of view, but in many, perhaps most, cases, this does still not explain why the disability occurred in the case of that particular child. A potentially powerful study would be to explore the narratives of parents of children with developmental communication disabilities. Understanding the stories of these parents might reveal understandings and misunderstandings and point to directions for parental education and counseling. Furthermore, the story that the parent tells about the child's communication disability will in some way, implicitly or explicitly, be part of the child's social context and be part of how the child learns to explain and live with his or her own disability.

People living with dysfluency might serve as a particularly interesting starting point in such a line of investigation, because there are well-organized self-help groups that range through the life span, and there are many published stories from which to cull information on their views of dysfluency. Kathard (2001) has argued well for taking a social constructionist position and incorporating the life narratives of individuals who stutter into our professional stance.

Adults who experience the abrupt onset of a communication disorder sometimes have a very specific medical diagnosis or explanation for what has occurred. But the medical diagnosis is not always sufficient. I remember a client of mine who had experienced a stroke with aphasia. In telling me his story, he ran down the list of risk factors for stroke. "Blood pressure? No! Cholesterol? No! Exercise? Yes! Smoking? No! Drinking? No! Mother-father? No! And young! Why, why, why?" he asked. No one could explain why a man in his early 40s with no obvious risk factors had experienced the devastating stroke that left him with aphasia and hemiparesis. And he had also not found an explanation that satisfied him, at least at that point.

Some explanations that clients tell about their disability might be in error—either because they were misinformed or because of some other personal or psychological motivation. Take for example a client of mine who also had stroke and aphasia. When asked about what he wanted to accomplish in a course of speech-language therapy, he insisted that what he really needed to improve his speech was physical therapy for his hemiparetic arm and leg. This gentleman, who at that point was 2 years post-stroke, had been well informed by a variety of health care professionals about stroke and the cause of his aphasia and hemiparesis. It seemed as though, for him, the hemiparesis was the visible disabling condition, and he was convinced that improving his arm and leg function would result in an improved language condition as well. Or perhaps his more visible disability was more important to him; if his arm and leg were improved, no one seeing him on the street would know that he was disabled or had experienced a stroke. His narrative about his problems and his own priorities were particularly revealing and also affected rehabilitation planning.

Other types of knowledge, besides just explanations for the onset of illness or disability, can also be revealed in illness narratives (Stern & Kirmayer, 2004). Knowledge about how an illness typically occurs or progresses and whether one's own illness or disability is usual or unusual can also be revealed in narratives. One time, when a client was talking about his hopes and dreams for the future, he tearfully told me that it was difficult to talk about the future because he was worried that his nonprogressive aphasia was going to get worse. It was not until that moment that I realized that this client had not yet formed a factual understanding of the relative stability of chronic aphasia due to stroke. He had understood that he had lost communication abilities, and fully expected to continue losing more.

Of course, knowledge about an illness or disability is a dynamic process. When facts are given about a traumatic event like an illness or disability, it is not reasonable to expect that hearing the facts one day will result in immediately being able to assimilate those facts into one's personal narrative the next day. It may take the retelling and reconstruction of one's narrative several times with many different conversational partners to fully integrate even medical facts into one's personal view of what has happened. Information that we provide as speech-language pathologists about the nature of communication disabilities often needs to be repeated in various ways, and clients and their families given the opportunity to tell their own narratives incorporating this information on multiple occasions.

To illustrate this point, consider the case of older adults living in an independent-living community who participated in a writing lab/journaling experience. These individuals were asked to write about a recent traumatic event or loss in their lives. Each participant wrote about the same experience over the course of three different sessions. The first writing session tended to be a factual account of the event. Accounts then become more focused on personal reactions and coping strategies and in particular on meaning-making across the series of writing sessions (Caplan, Haslett, & Burleson, 2005). It appears that there is a purpose to the multiple retelling of illness narratives; incorporating facts into one's life narrative and the meaning of the illness takes time and repetition.

In some cases, illness narratives can reveal the length of time it takes for patients to cope and adapt effectively, or rather, the amount of time it takes for patients to feel that they have coped or adapted effectively. In the case of atopic dermatitis with an onset in childhood, one study suggested that it took about 30 to 50 years for individuals to fully gather information about the disease and symptom management, and to develop effective social strategies around the illness (Diamond, 2005). The author suggested that this was due to a lack of access to total information; patients reported struggling to find information, and when they did it was in a piecemeal manner. It was also observed that self-management of any chronic disability is dependent on a certain degree of psychosocial maturity and thus is linked to an age-related developmental sequence. For self-management and coping to fully evolve, individuals must become proactive, learn stress reduction techniques, find social support, and overcome a sense of social isolation.

Illness narratives help us understand not only how people understand their own disabilities, but demonstrate the details of how one copes with living with a disability. The process of coping intersects with one's social life and relationships, and thus has a social presentation. But there is also a private aspect of coping that is played out in the daily minutiae of life, and this can be shown in narrative in a unique way. I always knew that individuals with hemiparesis had to learn adaptive strategies for getting dressed, but it was not until the day that a group of women clients told me stories about what they had gone through to learn to snap their bras on one-handed that I fully confronted in my mind's eye the daily challenge of getting dressed after hemiparesis.

A characteristic common to almost all chronic disabilities, including chronic communication disorders, is the fluctuating or inconsistent nature of symptoms and abilities. This inconsistency in ability from one day to the next or from one minute to another assaults our expectations and plans for the months or the day ahead, or even just our hopes for the current conversation. Just as illness can be considered an abrupt disruption to one's life narrative, so can inconsistency of symptoms or abilities be a brutal disruption to one's daily life. Narratives have been used as a means for understanding how inconsistency of symptoms affects social life and the construction of one's life narrative.

In a recent study, 10 individuals with unseen chronic illnesses related stories about how the inconsistency of symptoms and abilities and the expectation of consistency affected their own perceptions and their role in the workplace (Vickers, 2003). In this case, *unseen chronic illness* was defined as any long-standing incurable illness that did not have visible signs to colleagues. The participants themselves related expectations that they would be able to perform consistently at their jobs, as well as anecdotes indicating the same expectation from their work colleagues. The work life narratives revealed their disappointment with their inability to meet these expectations due to their chronic illnesses. The author observes that the mismatch between expectations for consistent performance and an inherent inconsistency that is part of the chronic illness may make coping with the disability more challenging than if allowance was made for fluctuating abilities.

Fluctuating symptoms are a hallmark of another condition, dementia due to Alzheimer's disease. Phinney (2002) conducted in-depth interviews and participant observation of nine adults with mild-to-moderate dementia of the Alzheimer's type and their families. Fluctuating cognitive abilities affected the individual's ability to formulate a cohesive illness narrative, because the experience or perceptions of certain symptoms were vague or absent at times. Thus it is difficult for individuals with dementia to create a meaningful narrative about what is happening to them. As the condition progresses, family members take on more of the storytelling and the narrative becomes a joint narrative. Eventually, the narrative may become a chaos narrative. The incorporation of narrative, identity, and coping in relation to dementia has been very thoroughly explored in a text by Hughes, Louw, & Sabat (2006).

Narratives reveal the details of how individuals cope with challenging and unexpected circumstances, and link one's identity with current circumstances surrounding the illness or disability. For example, breast cancer narratives are a means of redefining the self and reconnecting oneself. Narrative is characterized as both the process and the product of reestablishing identity after illness (Ford & Christman, 2005). An important part of this narrative process is the storytelling act and the selection of metaphors for creating meaning from the disability. Narratives from 16 women living with multiple sclerosis reveal a range of metaphors and meaning-making in accommodating to the inconsistencies of their illness in their everyday home and work lives (Wright-St. Clair, 2003).

The opportunity to tell your own illness narrative can produce beneficial effects. The outcomes of a cancer-related storytelling workshop were collected and analyzed by Chelf, Deshler, Hillman, and Durazo-Arvizu (2000). In this workshop, cancer patients were invited to come and hear a story presented by a professional storyteller. The workshop attendees then broke out into groups and told their own stories within smaller group settings. Six months later, a follow-up survey was sent out to the participants and a response rate of 70% was achieved. Respondents were generally positive and agreed that storytelling was effective for developing coping strategies. In particular, a large majority of the respondents indicated that storytelling was an effective means to transmit information, but that it also instilled hope and contributed to a sense of community among the cancer patients in attendance.

Illness narratives of individuals living with chronic disabilities can reveal general themes that have the potential to affect professional service options. From a set of personal narratives of individuals living with chronic disability, McColl (2003) identified four main themes. First, each narrative portrayed the emotional reaction to the initial diagnosis. The author discusses these in terms of "peak experiences," but one could also consider these "self-defining moments." Second, stress was discussed in the narratives as it was linked to experiencing symptoms or as it related to overall coping ability. All of the narratives identified their view of death as relating to their view of life, and this in turn led to the meaning that had been ascribed to the illness as a part of their lives. Two of the individuals providing narratives in this study described this as their "philosophy of life." Finding meaning in the disability experience has been classified by others as a part of the development of coping strategies (Lee & Poole, 2005).

Recently, I reviewed the published personal narratives of adults living with aphasia due to stroke to answer the question, "What does it take to live successfully with aphasia after stroke?" (Hinckley, 2006). Four main themes emerged from the reviewed narratives in response to this question. First, social support was identified within the narratives as critical to living successfully. Second, most of the narratives included a description of an adaptation of identity. The narratives also emphasized the importance of looking to the future and setting new goals. Finally, the narratives described the importance of taking control of one's own continued communication improvement. All of the narratives are manifest forms of meaning-making: figuring out what the onset of a communication disorder means in their lives, and what their lives mean now that they are living with a communication disorder.

Illness narratives are really life narratives in which an illness or disability is foregrounded. It's like telling a story about six people sitting in a waiting room. You can tell an overall story, or you can tell the story from the point of view of any of the six people. You get a different perspective in each case, but it is still a story about sitting in a waiting room. Thus illness narratives help us to recreate identity after illness or disability strikes, help us connect to others, and empower us to become active agents in the health care process. Listening to illness narratives has potentially healing effects for the individual with the illness. Professionals and researchers who listen to illness narratives can be shown how individuals understand their disability culturally and personally, how they cope, and how they manage their daily lives.

STUDY/DISCUSSION QUESTIONS AND ACTIVITIES

1. Listen for an illness narrative from a family member or friend. It could be an illness narrative about a recent cold or flu, or about something much more serious. What form does it take? What scenes are included? Is there detail about the onset of the illness and its course? Duration? Emotional reactions to the illness?

2. Review the case history given to you by one of your clients—either one you have recorded or from memory. What elements were included? Which ones did you probe for? What metaphors or illustrations did the client select to tell you? What might the way in which the client tells the story suggest to you about the life meaning the client is ascribing to the communication disorder?

6

Communication Disorders and Narrative

OVERVIEW

The study of narrative in speech-language pathology mostly focuses on how narrative reflects the interaction of cognition and language, narrative assessment tools and techniques, and interventions that generalize to narrative or are specifically targeted on narrative abilities. Another important aspect of narrative is its relation to personal and social identity. Directions for pursuing other aspects of narrative among those with communication disorders are suggested.

LEARNING OBJECTIVES

At the end of this chapter, the reader will be able to:

1. Identify two current, general approaches to narrative in speech-language pathology.

2. List three ways that narrative can be affected by various communication disorders.

3. Describe two intervention techniques specifically designed to improve narrative or personal narrative.

4. Discuss one way in which our view of narrative in communication disorders could be expanded in the practice of speech-language pathology.

The Study of Narrative in Communication Disorders

The study of narrative has attracted the attention of researchers and clinicians in speech-language pathology as well as other disciplines over the last couple of decades. Narrative has been described as entailing the following steps:

> (a) integrating a variety of themes with characters' motives and internal responses, (b) interweaving the content with socially appropriate and logical arguments for plans and outcomes, (c) molding that content into a language form that coherently realizes the narrative's communicative function, and (d) monitoring all of the above to produce the desired effect on the intended recipient (Liles, 1993, p. 871).

Each episode within a narrative discourse has identifiable components, including the setting, initiating event, internal response, plan, consequences, and reactions that are required to produce a grammatically well-formed narrative discourse (Caspari & Parkinson, 2000; Ulatowska & Bond, 1983). The events recounted can be real, such as recounting an experience, or imagined, such as a story retell. The intricate linkages between narrative structure and content with the context make it a sensitive and fertile genre for exploring how language intersects with cognition, social relationships, and culture.

Typical Approaches to Narrative in Communication Disorders

In speech-language pathology we have applied and investigated theoretical models of narrative from other domains such as social and cognitive psychology and linguistics, extending these research areas to the specific agenda of our field. Thus our own literature addresses narrative as an index of development across the life span, from the emergence of narrative as a communicative form in early childhood through progression to its forms, content, and uses in older adulthood. We have studied the potential differences and similarities in narrative between children and adults without communication disorders and those who do have communication disorders. Narrative has been a context in which the interplay of cognition and language can be explored. The ability to distinguish between normal narrative skills and those associated with communication disorders has led to the development of various assessment tools. Finally, we have used narrative as a point of intervention, an intervention technique, and an outcome measure for intervention efforts.

Narrative has been compared to other genres, determining how context affects different genres. Context effects within the same genre have also been a focus of research effort, such as comparing story retelling with story generation. Characteristics of the listener have also been manipulated to observe changes in narrative. Narrative has been viewed as an index of cognitive and social development, by relating measures of cognitive ability such as nonverbal intelligence measures with narratives. The text itself and the use of language across sentences have been analyzed through measure of coherence.

Thus the study of narrative in communication disorders can be broadly summarized as addressing three major areas. First are the internal characteristics of the group of interest; how language abilities (including semantic abilities and narrative structure) and cognitive abilities relate to narrative. Second is an interest in the context of the narrative, including the purpose, topic and content, and listener characteristics. Third is how the narrative itself is formed, including coherence and appropriate world knowledge to create logical progressions and outcomes within the narrative. A fourth potential dimension of narrative—a holistic view that relates narrative to global issues of identity, and to the context of a speech-language pathology session itself—has been little investigated. The purpose of this chapter is to provide a general overview of what is known about narrative in communication disorders, and to use this to point to additional aspects of narrative deserving of attention in our field.

Current Knowledge of Narrative in Communication Disorders

The following section broadly summarizes the conclusions and directions of narrative research within speech-language pathology. This is not meant as a comprehensive review, but rather a sampling of studies of narrative in communication disorders. The purpose of this section is to provide a starting point for a discussion of additional applications of narrative in the field of speech-language pathology as it pertains to our clients with communication disorders. Of course, new research is evolving and being published every day, so this brief overview should be considered a window into the state of the narrative literature.

Normally developing children begin to use simple narratives and logical associations by the age of 2½ years or 3 years. The complexity and completeness of the narrative structure itself gradually increases over the next couple of years. There appears to be a sudden spurt in the complexity of narrative development around the age of 5 years. By 6 years, the basic and complete, adultlike narrative structure is observed. After age 6 years, coherence, semantic abilities and relations, and narrative complexity continue to increase through later childhood years (for a review, see Liles, 1993).

Even among children with brain injury, the period between 5 and 7 years of age is a period of rapid growth in narrative abilities (Hemphill, Feldman, & Camp, 1994). Children with brain injury produce shorter narratives and are more likely to produce irrelevant or tangential information in their narratives. These children also have difficulty producing different genres of discourse, but characteristic genre features develop steadily between the ages of 5 and 7 years among children with or without brain injury.

Self-assessment of narrative abilities appears to improve with children's age. Kadaravek, Gillam, Ukrainetz, Justice, & Eisenberg (2004) found that children aged 10 to 12 years were more accurate than younger children at rating whether their narratives were a "good story" or not. They also observed that normally developing children who told poorer stories were less accurate in their self-ratings and were more likely to overestimate their own narratives. Finally, in their sample of 401 children, boys were more likely to overestimate their narrative ability than girls.

Children with language impairment show differences in narrative ability compared to typically developing children. When children are asked to generate a narrative to a wordless picture book, some studies have not observed global structure differences in narratives between children with language impairment and typically developing children (Norbury & Bishop, 2003). Other work has shown differences between children with language impairments and typically developing children on dimensions of topic maintenance, event sequencing, explicitness, referencing, cohesion, and fluency (Bliss, McCabe, & Miranda, 1998; Liles, 1985). Children who use augmentative and alternative communication due to speech difficulties as a result of cerebral palsy may also show difficulties with narrative and discourse organization (Soto & Harman, 2006).

Children who stutter have not been observed to demonstrate any difference in narrative abilities compared to children who do not stutter (Trautman, Healey, & Brown, 1999). There does not seem to be any evidence that children or adults with speech disorders and no language or cognitive impairment demonstrate any differences in narrative ability compared to those without speech, language, or cognitive disorders.

Among normally aging adults, some age-related changes in narrative production have been observed. When narratives are told from picture stimuli, older adults produce a greater quantity of output, less density of informational content, less tightly coherent narratives, and more irrelevant output than middle-aged adults (Juncos-Rabadan, Pereiro, & Rodriguez, 2005).

The relative contributions of language abilities and cognitive abilities to narrative production are sometimes more clearly studied in adult clinical populations, in whom we assume completed narrative development prior to injury and whose language and/or cognitive-linguistic disorder can be relatively easily identified, at least in relation to etiology. Doyle, Tsironas, Goda, & Kalinyak (1996) stated that discourse requires the use of strategies such as organization, selection of items to include or exclude, deductive thinking, and drawing conclusions. The cognitive processes important for discourse production include integration and organization of information, problem-solving, memory, word retrieval, inference, orientation, and attention (Cherney, 1998; Halper, Cherney, & Miller, 1991; Tompkins, 1995).

Adults with aphasia due to left hemisphere stroke or other focal injury produce narratives that are generally intact in terms of the basic structure. Ulatowska, Allard, Reyes, Ford, and Chapman (1992) found the macrostructure of speakers with aphasia to be comparable to normal speakers'. They examined the effectiveness of using role-playing situations to elicit discourse. Their interest in role-playing was to determine if script knowledge is preserved in speakers with aphasia. The role-plays were centered on dissatisfaction with a product or service. Variables such as the number of words, T-units, turns, and script knowledge were counted, and were compared to a normal subject control group. They found that the speakers with aphasia produced fewer T-units, with fewer clauses per T-unit, and fewer words. However, when comparing the discourse at the script level, topic structure and script maintenance were comparable in the aphasic and normal speakers.

Ulatowska, North, and Macaluso-Haynes (1981) compared the discourse of speakers with and without aphasia, and showed that the discourse produced by the speakers with aphasia included all the essential components of an episode, i.e., the settings, consequences, and reactions. The participants in this study were asked to give a self-generated account of a memorable experience, tell a story about a cat elicited with the help of sequence pictures, and retell a story about a rooster immediately following a reading of the story. The narratives also showed a preservation of the chronological sequence of events. There was a reduction in the complexity of language, with fewer words produced and less embedding and fewer clauses.

Linguistic aspects of narrative are affected by aphasia, such as cohesion, reference, and informativeness (Chapman, Highley, &

Thompson, 1998; Joanette, Lecours, Lepage, & Lamoureux, 1983; Nicholas & Brookshire, 1993; Ulatowska, Doyel, Stern, & Haynes, 1983; Yorkston & Beukelman, 1980). For example, Doyle, Tsironas, Goda, & Kalinyak. (1996) studied the connected speech of 25 adults with aphasia using ratings of informativeness, as judged by 11 unfamiliar listeners. They then compared these ratings with the measures obtained using correct information units (CIUs). They found an inverse relationship between the severity of aphasia and the amount of information conveyed by using the CIU when analyzing discourse. An increase in the number of CIUs was found to be a good predictor of the judgments of informativeness.

De Roo, Kolk, and Hofstede (2002) studied 13 individuals with Broca's aphasia using picture descriptions. They found that speakers with aphasia typically omit free grammatical morphemes such as determiners, pronouns, preposition, and auxiliaries. They further stated that tense inflection, verbal agreement, and number and gender markings on nouns and adjectives are omitted or substituted. Syntactic simplification is also seen, with utterances consisting of simple declaratives that are missing relative and subordinate clauses with very little subordination present, with reduced complexity of the language. De Roo and colleagues also concluded that speakers with aphasia produce more verbless constructions than normal speakers.

Saffran, Berndt, and Schwartz (1989) devised a system to quantify sentence production by analyzing lexical types such as open class words, nouns, determiners, pronouns, and verbs, taking into account the inflection of the verb. They also looked at sentences, requiring at least minimal evidence of constituents such as noun + verb, noun + copula + adjective, or prepositional phrase. They examined the number of embeddings in each sentence, morphological content, and structural complexity. This study included participants with chronic aphasia and a group of normal controls. The results indicated that the sentences of the speakers with chronic aphasia were structurally simple, with very little embedding or elaboration. They also found a significant reduction in the use of grammatical morphemes, a marked reduction in verb inflection, and omission of determiners when compared to the normal speakers.

Discourse production of adults with right hemisphere disorder (RHD) due to stroke or other focal lesions has been reported to be disrupted, verbose, and tangential with abrupt topic shifting

(Brownell & Martino, 1998; Gainotti, Caltagironi, & Miceli, 1983; Joanette, Goulet, Ska, & Nespoulous, 1986; Myers, 1993: 1997) and differentiated from the discourse of adults with aphasia due to left hemisphere damage (Bloom, 1994). Trupe and Hillis (1985) reported the verbal production of adults with RHD was literal, with primary focus on minute, extraneous detail of picture description rather than integration of the picture as a whole. Individuals with RHD may show impairments with the integration of information (Delis, Wapner, Gardner, & Moses, Jr., 1983; Hough & Pierce, 1993; Myers, 1993), and they may also have significant problems with discourse comprehension and production (Davis, O'Neill-Pirozzi, & Coon, 1997; McDonald, 2000). In some cases, the features of disorganization apparent in the discourse of individuals with RHD have been linked to difficulties with unilateral visual neglect (Cherney, Drimmer, & Halper, 1997) or other visuospatial impairment (Moya, Benowitz, Levine, & Finklestein, 1986).

Adults who have sustained traumatic brain injury (TBI) demonstrate difficulty with coherence and organization of semantic-syntactic relationships in narrative (Coelho, 2002; Mentis & Prutting, 1987; Stout, Yorkston, & Pimentel, 2000). Generally, adults with TBI show reductions in fluency and the rate of information provided, or information efficiency. In both a story retelling and story generation contexts, adults with TBI produce fewer propositions per T-unit, or less propositional complexity, than adults without TBI (Coelho, Grela, Corso, Gamble, & Feinn, 2005). Adults with TBI, like adults with right hemisphere dysfunction and children with TBI, are more likely to provide irrelevant or tangential information in narratives (McDonald, 1993). Children with TBI, similarly, produce much less fluent narratives than same-aged peers without TBI, like adults with TBI (Biddle, McCabe, & Bliss, 1996). They are not sensitive to the listener and aberrant patterns of the use of contingent queries have been observed (Prince, Haynes, & Haak, 2002). These discourse impairments are likely to persist for years after brain injury (Snow, Douglas, & Ponsford, 1998).

Adults with dementia share some discourse similarities with adults with right hemisphere brain injury, but also demonstrate particular differences (Cherney & Canter, 1993). Adults with dementia of the Alzheimer's type demonstrate shorter utterance length and reduced content in narratives elicited with pictures or otherwise (Ehrlich, Obler, & Clark, 1997). In this case, reduced content was observed through fewer propositions and lexical items used in the narratives. Particular changes in semantic and syntactic production in discourse are not limited to dementia associated with Alzheimer's, but have also been observed in Huntington's and Parkinson's diseases (Murray, 2000). A particular feature of discourse in dementia is a deterioration of semantic organization and coherence. This extends to an inability to participate fully in extended conversations and other aspects of discourse. Certain personal stories or other, perhaps overtold, narratives are sometimes retained as units for some time into the progression of the disease (Guendouzi & Muller, 2006). Narrative discourse and personal narratives are now being used to explore how dementia relates to the continuity or disorganization of the self and relationships to important others (Hughes, Louw, & Sabat, 2006).

Narrative develops predictably over the course of the life span. Children begin with their first personal narratives about an event during the day and develop to more complex structures and increased informativeness. As adults age, narrative production may become longer with less highly relevant information (North, Ulatowska, Macaluso-Haynes, & Bell, 1986). So, we can identify narrative production abilities that are more or less consistent with normally developing age peers.

Language or cognitive-linguistic disorder at any age affects the ability to produce narratives. Changes in informativeness, fluency, cohesion, and relevance are observed across several different clinical populations. These observations support the notion that narrative requires an integration of language and cognitive abilities, including world and social knowledge, and sensitivity to context, including listener characteristics.

The elicitation technique of the narrative does affect the complexity of semantic-syntactic forms produced. It has been argued by some that personal narrative is the most highly relevant to everyday living. Story retelling appears to reduce the cognitive-linguistic load compared to story generation. The presence of visual stimuli in either case seems to increase the requirement for visual-spatial processing while increasing the comparability of the context from which each individual produces the narrative. Providing the moral in a fable and completing proverb interpretation tasks are sensitive to the differences between African-American adults with aphasia and African-American adults without aphasia (Ulatowska et al.,

2001); these seem to be discourse tasks that are particularly useful for adults.

Finally, narrative can be used as a measure of change in relation to intervention efforts, or as a target of intervention itself. This will be reviewed further in a separate section.

Special Aspects of Narrative

Narrative discourse is special because it is one form that is typically used multiple times during the day every day by most people. Telling stories of what has happened to us during the day or what might happen is an important part of our social fabric. Everyday narrative communicates to others who we are; as discussed in Chapter 1, telling stories about ourselves reflects connections to our culture while distinguishing us as individuals. We also know that successful, coherent narrative is dependent on sufficient language, cognitive, emotional, and social knowledge resources. Narrative reveals more than just the interaction of certain language and cognitive skills; it positions the individual within her immediate culture and social relationships.

Communication disorders, and in particular language disorders, interact with emotional, social, and cognitive development. Thus individuals with at least some types of communication disorders who have difficulties with narrative are at risk for social, emotional, and cognitive difficulties as well. Indeed, children with behavioral difficulties are often overlooked or undiagnosed in relation to their language impairments, including pragmatic abilities (Cross, 1999).

Narrative, along with other discourse abilities, provides a means to independence and social interaction. In an interview study of an individual with autism who became a successful user of facilitated communication and then independent typing, Rubin and coresearchers explain how participation in social communication interacts with a developing sense of identity, independence, and participation in the world (Rubin et al., 2001). Rubin and colleagues poignantly suggest that successful communication at the social discourse level enables the individual with a disability to be perceived differently, to share a mental existence with others that may otherwise be unknown and therefore assumed to be nonexistent.

What speech-language pathologists know about narrative in relation to various communication disorders is relevant to our clients' emotional-behavioral development, sense of self, and social relationships. Narrative in particular, compared to other discourse genres, deserves attention because it is so prominent in typical everyday life. Research efforts in our field show that narrative is a fertile ground as a target of intervention and an intervention outcome. A new direction for our field, however, is to expand our view of narrative to consider how narrative abilities affect the individual's sense of self, well-being, and social development.

Personal Narrative Is Different from Other Genres

Beginning with toddlers and through the rest of the life course, narrative and in particular personal narrative is pervasive. From a sample of 90 hours of conversation between three 5-year-old children over a period of 18 months, it was observed that 52% of all narratives were personal anecdotes. Seventy percent of all of the conversational narratives produced by these young children communicated personal events (Preece, 1987).

As children mature and enter adolescence, the need for conversational abilities increases and expands to include the use of more complex language forms such as sarcasm and metaphor (Brinton, Robinson, & Fujiki, 2004; Brinton & Fujiki, 2002; Brinton, Fujiki, & Highee, 1998; Fujiki, Brinton, & Todd, 1996; Craig & Washington, 1993). Structural language impairments affect the ability to access and learn academic information and thus impact academic achievement. Similarly, language impairments affect access to and development of social relationships, thus impacting behavior, social achievement, and personal success.

Towards the end of the life course, personal narrative extends not only to events of the day but to reminiscing about previous life events and making sense of one's life story. I once heard the story of a grandfather with his grandchildren gathered around him in the evening, looking down at his hand. And, looking at the lines in his hand, he told stories of the adventures of his life. Personal narrative continues to be a critical and predominant aspect of conversation and social life.

Personal familiarity influences how a narrative is produced. Speech-language pathologists in particular are attentive to this when assessing narrative abilities. Children may be reluctant or even unable to relate a narrative that is not familiar or personally relevant. Older adults, without aphasia or with aphasia, are more likely to include more action and resolution clauses in their retelling of a familiar story than when the story is not personally familiar (Li, Williams, & Della Volpe, 1995). When the listener is familiar with the story, adults with and without aphasia are more likely to include more information about the setting of the story (Li, Williams, & Della Volpe, 1995).

Preschool children with language impairment show patterns of differences when asked to perform in either conversational or narrative tasks (Wagner, Nettelbladt, Sahlen, & Nilholm, 2000). The narrative condition facilitates the production of mean length of utterance in words, phrasal expansions, and grammatical morphemes per utterance. Conversation enhances intelligibility, fluency, and complexity of verb forms.

Narrative requires the ability to take another's perspective and to manipulate concepts about mental states and inferred intention. The inability to perform perspective-taking and to imagine others' mental states under various conditions relates ultimately to narrative performance. The "capacity to reason about covert mental states" is referred to as *theory of mind* (ToM) (Peterson & Slaughter, 2006, p. 151). Children with autism, as well as children who are deaf or who have hearing impairment, are delayed in their development of theory of mind as measured by standard false belief tasks. Peterson and Slaughter (2006) used standard false belief tasks, such as showing a child a scenario in which a girl doll hid a marble in one location and leaves; a boy doll comes and moves the marble to a second location, and the child is asked "Where will the girl look for her marble?" In a series of two studies with deaf children matched to typically developing hearing children, Peterson and Slaughter (2006) observed a strong relationship between performances on standard false belief tasks and the production of mental state vocabulary during narration of a wordless picture book. It appears that, in the case of autism, children are limited in their linguistic and cognitive abilities to benefit from social conversation at an early age that would facilitate the development of ToM. Deaf children, particularly those being raised by hearing parents with limited or no signing skills, are also delayed in their development of ToM, apparently due to the communicative barriers they experience early in their childhood, which limits their exposure to typical conversation and narrative about internal states.

In fact, Peterson and Slaughter's (2006) data suggested that there was a consistent sequence of development in relation to narrative performance and false belief task performance for both hearing and deaf children. First, children use visible mental state terms in their narratives, but fail false belief tasks. Next, children add to visible mental state terms mention of cognitive states, and then mention of inner states during narrative. Finally, narratives include affective, perceptual, and cognitive state terms along with success on false belief tasks. These observations support the strong relationship between narrative abilities, theory of mind, linguistic-cognitive development, and ultimately social relationships.

Performance differences are observed among adults and children with TBI when they relate a personal narrative. The task involved the examiner relating a personal story, such as being stung by a bee or being involved in a car accident, and asking the participant if she had ever experienced something similar. This then elicits a personal narrative, the most common form of narrative, requiring the integration of social, cognitive, and language abilities (McCabe & Peterson, 1991). Adults and children with TBI tended to omit critical information and lack self-monitoring of the narrative produced, requiring the listener to make guesses and interpretations that remained unclear (Biddle et al., 1996). The observed difficulties with personal narratives among adults and children with TBI, compared to those without TBI, appeared to be related to executive function deficits including lack of planning and organization.

From the point of view of narrative assessment in speech-language pathology, using personally familiar narratives may provide different types of information in the course of an evaluation. Increased access to the episodic knowledge required for production of the narrative macrostructure in a personally familiar narrative condition could provide the speaker with strategies to increase the optional elements and elaborations in the production of discourse. On the other hand, relating a previously unfamiliar narrative with decreased demand for access to the episodic knowledge could provide the speaker with more efficient access to the lexical-semantic system, thus providing a clearer picture of that system during an assessment (Caspari & Parkinson, 2000; Ulatowska et al., 1992).

Personal narrative develops early in the life course and continues to be a prominent feature of social discourse throughout the life span. Different linguistic features may be elicited in personal narrative compared to other discourse genres, and this is an issue from the point of view of language assessment in speech-language pathology. But the ramifications of being able to adequately produce personal narrative are vast in relation to one's sense of identity and social relationships. Therefore, personal narrative is a critical discourse context deserving of attention by speech-language pathologists in assessment and intervention.

Narrative Is Amenable to Intervention

There are two general ways to think about affecting personal narrative through intervention. First, structural language impairments can be addressed via nonconversational techniques, and generalization may occur to conversational abilities. Second, conversation or personal narrative itself can be specifically and directly targeted in the intervention approach.

There is some evidence that, occasionally, conversational and narrative abilities improve as a result of intervention that targets specific language forms. In this case, intervention designed to improve semantic or syntactic abilities is spontaneously used successfully in social discourse. Among children with language and pragmatic impairments, conversational and narrative abilities improve, even after ceilings are reached on standardized tests (Adams, Lloyd, & Aldred, 2006). Impairments at the microstructural level may affect the organization of discourse due to the inability of speakers to retrieve the words and sentence forms needed to produce discourse. Among adults with aphasia, improvements in word-finding can be reflected in increases in content and efficiency of communication (Honda, Mitachi, & Watamori, 1999).

Correlations between standardized testing and measures of conversational or narrative performance have been observed. For example, performance on standardized aphasia batteries such as the Western Aphasia Battery (WAB) and the Porch Index of Communicative Ability (PICA) are correlated with performance on measures of functional communication such as the Communicative Abilities in Daily Living test (CADL) and measures of content production and efficiency (correct information units) (Ross & Wertz, 1999). Similarly, objective measures are related to listener perceptions and ratings (Doyle, Tsironas, Goda & Kalnyak, 1996). Standardized measures are often observed to relate to measures of discourse performance or listener perceptions of communication adequacy.

Although performance on standardized and more objective measures after a course of intervention targeting language forms may be related to conversational or narrative performance, these measures are not equivalent and cannot be substituted for one another (Ross & Wertz, 1999; Doyle, Tsironas, Goda, & Kalinyakm, 1996). Lyon et al. (1997) compared changes on measures of content and information in discourse to standardized test measures following a course of treatment. The results showed statistically significant gains in communication that were not detected on standardized measures. In this case, it was argued that the standardized measures were not specific or sensitive enough to measure the gains made in treatment.

At times targeting structural language elements in intervention may generalize to social discourse situations, but not always. Social discourse can be directly and specifically targeted during intervention with a view towards affect social communication behaviors and performances.

For example, discourse can serve as a medium for improving word finding (Stiegler & Hoffman, 2001). Within story-retelling tasks, picture-elicited narratives, and conversation, clinicians identified word-finding behaviors, facilitated their completion, and aided in the production of associated information as needed. This type of intervention was shown to produce positive results among three 9-year-old boys with language learning disability.

In an even more direct approach, Brinton, Robinson, and Fujiki (2004) describe a social communication intervention program for an adolescent male who had been receiving speech-language services for his language disability since the age of 5 years. By the time he entered junior high school his language disorder was significantly limiting his ability to function in social conversations and develop social relationships. A communication intervention was designed that centered around two main activities. One activity involved the client and his clinician actively reviewing video clips, either from movies or role-plays by other clinic personnel. In this activity the clinician focused the client on how each of the conversational partners might feel or react based on what was being said and occurring during the conversation. The second activity was dubbed "the conversation game" and emphasized the reciprocal nature of conversation. A hierarchy of targets was devised that gradually increased the number of comments, questions, and responses the client should produce in a conversation with the clinician.

At the end of a year of intervention, important improvements in this adolescent client's social life were observed. He was more successful in conversation with his family and also at school with his peers, and he began to enjoy social relationships at school, something that had previously been aversive for him. Although intervention focusing on structural language like vocabulary, word-finding, and grammatical forms improved academic achievement in this client's case, this type of intervention was not sufficient to facilitate appropriate social development, particularly in adolescence. This social communication intervention illustrates how directly targeting social discourse skills may be necessary above and beyond typical language targets.

Social stories are being used with children with autism as a means to improve their linguistic functioning in relation to social discourse and social relationships (see Silliman et al., 2003). In this technique, children are read stories about social situations in which the internal mental states of the characters in the story figure prominently. Scaffolding is offered by the clinician as the child responds to questions that facilitate integration of the social information and perspective-taking.

Conversational strategies have been directly targeted in some interventions designed for adults with aphasia and their conversational partners (e.g., Fox, Poulson, & Bowden, 2004; Hopper, Holland, & Rewega, 2002). In these approaches, the person with aphasia and her conversational partner both have goals to achieve in the course of the intervention, and the practice involves both of them with the clinician acting in the role of communication coach.

A conversational emphasis has also been observed to work well when improving conversational interaction of adults with dementia of the Alzheimer's type (DAT). In one study, Spilkin (2003) targeted turn-taking, topic management, and repair in the conversations of an adult with DAT and his caregiver. A memory book was featured as an assist to conversational success. As a result of a brief educational intervention, the caregiver perceived improvements in their ability to carry on conversations.

In a broader-scale study within a nursing home, nursing home residents and nursing assistants participated in an intervention designed to specifically target conversation including the use of memory books. Nursing home residents with dementia and nursing assistants were divided into two groups, one receiving the intervention and a control group. Conversational assessments after intervention showed an improvement in coherence and fewer empty phrases among the nursing home residents in the treatment group. Similarly, nursing assistants who participated in the treatment showed more facilitative strategies in conversation, including cueing and encouragement, than those staff members who had not participated in the intervention (Dijkstra, Bourgeois, Burgio, & Allen, 2002).

These are just a few examples of how narrative is affected either by targeting microstructural aspects of language in an intervention program, or by directly addressing specific conversational and social discourse skills, including narrative. The links between narrative and social-behavioral abilities is sufficiently strong that it has been suggested that narrative training be offered to teachers. Training teachers about narratives, in how to facilitate groups, and in improving the written and oral narratives of students with learning and behavioral difficulties may be an effective avenue for improving behavior through a narrative-based approach (Sage, 2005).

Narrative, Communication Disorders, and Identity

It is clear that narrative relates to social relationships in various ways. Hearing and participating in narratives within the family appears to foster the development of theory of mind, including perspective-taking and the understanding and manipulation of internal state terms. Social relationships are a key to normal development to adulthood, and later, narrative is the core of the maintenance of social relationships. In more recent years, speech-language pathologists have identified these relationships and sought to develop interventions that improve social communication and as a result the facilitation of social relationships among our clients. Language abilities and social-behavioral abilities meet at various points, but a frequently occurring interaction point is narrative.

The absence of narrative has been attributed to a perception of fragmented behavior, devoid of meaning. A parallel can be drawn between observations of what appears to be incoherent behavior and observations of machines using artificial intelligence. When observing artificial intelligence, observers are unable at times to create a narrative from the actions that artificial intelligences produce. Thus the observed behavior appears fragmented and devoid of contextualized meaning. It has been argued that what is needed in the future design of artificial intelligence is a narrative schema: adding the ability to project sequences of events linked through time (Mateas & Sengers, 2003). Adding the elements of narrative to an artificial intelligence (AI) design may increase coherence in series of actions and improve the interface between humans and AI machines.

Humans who do not have narrative ability may also be perceived as lacking coherence in their behaviors, and thus be perceived as mentally impaired. The inability of observers to form a coherent narrative from the behavior of schizophrenics may explain why their behavior is perceived as bizarre and fragmented. Such a narrative-based view could be extended to other behavioral disorders, potentially including autism. An individual with autistic behaviors may not seem to create a coherent narrative to others, thus preventing others around the individual from being able to understand or predict behavior.

Individuals with traumatic brain injury or right hemisphere disorder, whether children or adults, may produce irrelevant or tangential comments and have difficulty maintaining topic in conversation. Their narrative productions may lack intersentential and intrasentential cohesion and lack appropriate sequencing of events. These narrative impairments associated with their linguistic-cognitive status may lead to perceptions of incoherent behavior and disorganized thinking and prevent others from predicting their behavior. This may seriously hamper social relationships with caregivers and others in the environment, and prevent the development of new social relationships.

Adults with dementia and associated linguistic-cognitive impairments may also show difficulties with narrative. In the early and middle stages, adults with linguistic-cognitive impairments associated with dementia may have difficulty maintaining relevance and topic due to memory impairments, although they may be able to tell personal stories about past life events quite well. This may lead to the layperson's view that such an individual is living in the past and cannot relate to the present.

We know that narrative abilities relate to behavior, social skills, and the development of social relationships. From a narrative-based perspective, we can view others' perceptions of narrative abilities as creating a lack of coherence and sequential meaning to their behavior and ultimately to their capacities as individuals. A narrative-based approach emphasizes the role of narrative abilities in developing and maintaining social relationships.

Narrative abilities may affect more than social relationships; a lack of narrative ability may in fact affect one's own view of oneself, and the ability to maintain or create one's identity. Narrative can be conceptualized as a means by which we develop our own sense of identity; it is how we link events of the day and events of our lives cohesively. Thus the narrative abilities of our clients do not only affect their ability to maintain family relationships or develop friendships, but also affect their own ability to develop a sense of themselves, a sense of their own life story including potential future chapters and life events. Thus narrative abilities are also linked to planning and organizing, and this extends not just to the organization of one's homework assignments, but potentially and more holistically to the organization of thinking about one's own life.

It has been argued that impaired narrative ability, whether limited in development or newly impaired due to injury or disease, results in a loss of one's self and one's own identity. "Individuals who have lost the ability to construct narratives have lost their selves" (Young & Saver, 2001). Presumably the loss of narrative ability results in the loss of the maintenance of a coherent strand through past and current life events, and hinders the imagination of future life events (Sengers, 2000; 2003).

Children with autism, who do not have a sense of the other or the other's internal states, may not create a sense of their own self, either. Development of one's identity comes through social exchange and learning about similarities and differences between others' mental states and our own. Children with language and pragmatic impairments without autism experience at least a delay in developing social skills and social relationships, and may also be delayed in their development of their own sense of identity.

Individuals with dementia due to Korsakoff's or Alzheimer's who have lost the ability to tell cohesive narratives may have also lost a sense of themselves. It has been observed that, in the case of dementia, fluctuating cognitive abilities affect the individual's ability to tell a cohesive illness narrative (Phinney, 2002). It is likely that fluctuating cognitive abilities also affect, then, the ability to tell a cohesive narrative about one's own life course. Although past nuclear episodes may still be told relatively coherently, an overall story of one's life may well be affected by the cognitive-linguistic impairments associated with dementia.

A narrative-based approach to living with communication disorders focuses attention on social perceptions and identity. Such an approach may help to identify and prioritize intervention for those communication behaviors that particularly affect narrative and thus link to social relationships and a view of oneself. One individual, living with aphasia and writing about it, urged clinicians to help patients reconsider their sense of self beginning in the early stages of rehabilitation (Hall, 1961). Thinking holistically about individuals, perhaps through a narrative-based approach, must be maintained even while we develop a stricter sense of evidence-based practice.

Extending Our View of Narrative in Communication Disorders

At present, the bulk of the research and clinical work in the area of narrative in speech-language pathology has focused on identifying the relationships between certain cognitive-linguistic skills and narrative abilities. Some work in speech-language pathology has broadened its focus to show how narrative and other discourse skills should be targeted to facilitate the social development of the individual. What we lack so far is a true incorporation of a holistic view of people living with communication disorders into our theory building, hypothesis testing, and observational work. A narrative-based approach emphasizes such a holistic view by acknowledging global concepts like identity. The personal, social, and cultural milieu of the person living with a communication disorder should play a powerful part in the research and clinical agenda of speech-language pathologists.

Just such an argument has been presented by Kathard (2001), who suggests that the life experiences of people who stutter should contribute significantly to the development of theory of research and practice. Kathard argues that a conceptual shift is required in the ways speech-language pathologists develop and construct knowledge about communication disorders, and specifically, stuttering. A top-down approach to theory and practice development, in which theory comes from an isolated ivory tower and moves downward finally to application (to use a factory metaphor) seriously neglects critical and holistic views of the life experience of the communication disorder. Those who are living with any given communication disorder are experts in that experience. Their life experiences must not only be acknowledged but actively incorporated into the development of our professional knowledge base.

The life history narrative is one means by which we can access information about the lived experience of those with communication disorders, and we can develop a fuller view of how our actions and inactions as clinicians interact with their view of themselves and their life experiences. Kathard (2001) uses the life history of one person who stutters to show how stuttering was incorporated into his life but faded against other important life and political events in which the individual was involved.

Recently, I had occasion to review a set of published life and illness narratives written by people living with aphasia due to stroke (Hinckley, 2006). Several themes emerged from the review. One common theme among many of the publications was the incorporation of the aphasia into the individual's life, and the recognition that the aphasia was something to be continuously worked on and improved over time. This persistent desire to improve a perceived shortfall in communication abilities was set against a backdrop of newly developed and future life goals. Thus these individuals, experts on living successfully after stroke and aphasia, carried the present circumstance of aphasia into the development of their future life stories.

Narrative is more than just a discourse genre that relates to particular cognitive and linguistic functions. Narrative abilities on the part of our clients are necessary for their personal and social welfare. Our clients' narratives also inform us about their experience of living with a communication disorder. A narrative-based approach to practice in speech-language pathology widens our view of both how communication disorders affects all aspects of one's life and also how clinical practice has the potential to affect all aspects of our clients' lives.

STUDY/DISCUSSION QUESTIONS AND ACTIVITIES

1. Reflect on and discuss a recent clinical example of your own in which narrative abilities figured prominently. Position your recent experience with the current literature.
2. Describe one example of a narrative-based assessment or intervention that is not mentioned in this chapter.
3. Discuss how the presence of a communication disorder has affected the development of a life narrative of one of your clients.

Section III

Stories of a Clinical Life

"Adventures happen to people who know how to tell about them."

—Henry James

7

God and Truth

It was during my first year as a practicing clinician that Mark was admitted to the physical medicine and rehabilitation service at the teaching hospital where I had been lucky enough to get a fellowship position. Mark had been in a motor vehicle accident, and they had used the Jaws of Life to extricate him from the crumbled wreckage. They rushed him to the regional trauma hospital via helicopter—the one we usually referred to as Death Star, because of the high mortality rate associated with the patients who had to come to the hospital in this way.

Mark was a 28-year-old man, about the same age as I was at the time, who was married and who had not been drinking at the time of his accident. By all accounts, it was another car that had jumped across the median and hit his car head-on. He hadn't done anything to "deserve" his fate.

He was medically stabilized and quickly admitted to the rehabilitation service, where the treating physician sent out the referrals to physical therapy (PT), occupational therapy (OT), and speech pathology. When the referral came down towards the end of that day, all the other clinicians in speech pathology had full caseloads; and besides, it would be a great experience, they reasoned, for the new fellow to follow a case like this one from beginning to end. The referral read: "Traumatic Brain Injury—please evaluate and treat."

Dutifully, I called up to the rehab floor to arrange my first appointment with this new patient. It was set for the next morning, before physical therapy got in there and fatigued him. The next morning I headed upstairs to begin my evaluation of this new patient. I hadn't been at the process of being a speech pathologist long enough to not feel a little anxious about walking into a new patient's room. I knew he had a traumatic brain injury, and I knew how many different things that could mean in terms of the patient's behavior. I didn't know what I would find when I walked into that room. Would I handle the situation appropriately? Would I be able to do the right bedside assessments to come up with some idea of the patient's cognitive status? Would I make the kind of observations that my supervisor would ask me about?

I stopped at the nurse's station to look at the patient's chart. Mark's chart had a variety of lab tests, CT scan results, and other technical reports, but I spent most of my time reading the history and physical note that was written when he was admitted to the rehab service. It provided an overview of the accident and his injuries, and a very brief description of his behavior since then.

The CT scan results suggested that Mark had bilateral damage, to both left and right hemispheres, fairly typical for many TBI cases. Mark had also sustained many other injuries besides his TBI. He had bone fractures in three of his four extremities, and as a result he had been put into traction of various types. He had also broken his mandible.

I wasn't exactly sure what I was going to do for an assessment, as a speech-language pathologist, if my patient had his jaw wired shut and both arms in traction, limiting all usual forms of expressive communication. Well, I thought, if the patient can't participate, I will just monitor him every day until he can participate in something, and maybe pick up another patient to fill this time slot, when a new referral comes down later today.

I walked into Mark's room. Although I had seen the metal "halos" that patients with spinal cord injuries wear to stabilize their heads and necks, I hadn't seen the kind of pins and metal frames that he had around his arms and legs before. Emulating all of the other medical professionals who surrounded me, I worked hard not to notice or stare. In my best medical speech-language pathologist's voice, I smiled and said, "Hello, Mark, how are you today?" Mark opened his eyes wide, looking towards me, but not saying anything. "My name is Jackie Hinckley, and I'm the speech pathologist who will be working with you." I pressed on, wondering if some nurse somewhere could hear me and was secretly laughing, because I was trying to engage in a conversation with someone who was obviously incapable of responding. "What's your name? Do you know where you are?"

Mark wasn't able to reliably respond to any of this verbal stimulation, and mostly just moved his head around—the only part of his body that wasn't externally restricted. I put a note in the chart, indicating that the patient was functioning at Rancho Los Amigos Level III—Localized response, and that speech pathology would continue to assess and monitor.

Every day for a week or two I walked that route up to his room, doing a brief evaluation, and noting that he continued to be at the same functional level. I never met his wife, because she worked and only came in during the evenings. Whenever I was up on the same floor to see another patient, I found myself peeking in his room to see how he was doing, or asking the nurses how Mark was doing today.

After about a week or two of only moving his head around, things began to change. When I arrived in his room in the morning, right after OT and before PT, he was noticeably more specifically responsive to verbal stimulation, and in fact, he began to speak. Mark's first word was the same one he would utter perseveratively for another 3 or 4 weeks. It was a four-letter word, beginning with a labiodental. Because his jaw was still wired, that first phoneme wasn't really articulated clearly, but he was able to get the vowel sound and that last velar well enough for everyone on the ward to be clear about what he was saying. His voice had good quality and volume, which was good to know since he had been intubated early on. I went over Mark's memory book, showing him and saying aloud to him his name, where he was, and today's date, and showed him family pictures that had been left on his bedside table. To each of these efforts, the response was that same, misarticulated but clearly identifiable word.

I wrote a note in the chart that day saying that Mark had moved into Rancho Los Amigos Level IV—Confused/Agitated. Unlike other agitated patients, Mark didn't need to be restrained, because his multiple fractures and tractions functionally accomplished that. The only way he could release this agitation was verbally, with that one obscene word, yelled loudly, over and over and over again.

As tragic as this situation really was, and how horrible it must have been for his wife and two young children, the hospital staff had its own way of dealing with this situation. Every day I went in to administer my stimulation and orientation treatment, and every day I was greeted with that same lovely word. Finally, nurses and other therapists started asking me, "Jackie, you're the speech pathologist, can't you teach him another word?" Shortly thereafter, Mark added a new cuss word to his repertoire, bringing the total up to two. This one was a little less offensive, and although I had nothing whatsoever to do with Mark's new verbal behavior, I jokingly took every bit of credit for it that I could.

During this period I did finally meet Mark's wife, who tearfully asked me why her husband could only say cuss words. I tried to explain what a brain injury was, and the stages of healing that we could expect him to go through, and that this stage, agitation, was just one of those that would pass eventually (I hoped). She told me that she could not bring their young sons to see their father like this, but was looking forward to the day when he would be better and the boys could come to see Daddy.

The agitation started to lessen, and Mark became able to respond to simple questions and commands at times, with short phrases. He was moving into Level V—Confused—Automatic. Each of our daily sessions consisted of reviewing orientation information, looking at family photos, and sometimes doing other simple language tasks, like following simple commands, or naming pictures. These last activities were to help track Mark's cognitive and linguistic abilities as he progressed through the stages of recovery from brain injury.

At this point I was feeling very comfortable in my ability to manage Mark's case. I had, apparently, assessed him adequately considering all of his limitations so far, or so my supervisor confirmed, and the other rehab professionals on his team seemed satisfied with my input at team meetings. Mark had even afforded me an occasion to get to know some of the other nurses and staff on the rehab ward a bit better, what with all those jokes about teaching him new words. And now that he was better able to respond, at least to simple tasks, there were more things I could try with him, which overall made me feel more comfortable and competent.

Weeks had gone by and many of Mark's fractures were healing. Some of the tractions and frames on his extremities were changed or removed, and even his jaw was released from its limitations. Unfortunately, the removal of the wires from his jaw did not improve his ability to speak meaningfully or appropriately at all times, like his wife had hoped. However, it did mean that Mark could get up in a wheelchair, and pretty soon he could be wheeled down to the clinic for appointments in my office.

Like most hospital speech-language pathologists, and especially fellows, my office space was small. It was a fairly new hospital, though, and I had a built-in desk and a separate table that I used for treatment. I managed to arrange an optimal morning appointment time, and since transportation for the patients was sometimes unreliable, I went up to get Mark and wheel him down for the appointment myself. Because he still had one leg and arm extended in semitraction, it was difficult to fit him all the way under the table. So I pushed him into my office as far as I could, but it wasn't far enough to be able to shut the door. I pushed past him to the desk side of the table. Now we were really able to do some therapeutic activities in earnest, there in the office with a table to write on, a more conducive environment than bedside.

I began with doing some basic tasks that would contribute to the continual assessment of Mark's cognitive and linguistic abilities. He was still disoriented, although he was able to say his name and starting inconsistently to recognize that he was in the hospital because of an accident. Because I transported Mark down to my office myself each morning, I was able to make sure that he had his memory book with him, and we were able to review his orientation information, review entries from the previous day, and write summaries of what we did in our sessions.

In contrast to the early days of Mark's hospitalization, I was really enjoying working with him now. In the beginning, seeing Mark was a source of some nervousness for me, because I wasn't very confident about treating lower level patients yet. Now I felt that I had a routine going with Mark, one that seemed to be meeting with everyone's approval, and Mark and I seemed to have a rhythm and rapport going that made my appointment with him each morning seem like a productive one.

A couple more weeks of these office appointments and Mark was able to indicate his name, where he was, who I was, and what he was doing in the hospital. Of course, he didn't really remember who I was the way someone else would. He would look at me, look at his schedule, see me opening his memory book, and say something like, "You must be my speech therapist." But he knew I was a therapist, and that this person across the table from him wearing a white lab coat was intending to help him with problems that he was only vaguely beginning to appreciate.

Mark was beginning to do well enough to have visits with his whole family, kids included, on the weekends, and these visits seem to collectively trigger more insight. Particularly on Mondays after these visits, Mark engaged in more and more appropriate conversation with me at the beginning of our therapy session. During these conversational sessions, I encouraged Mark to ask me questions as well. When I asked him what he did the day before, and he answered me, I would cue him, saying "How about asking me what I did last night?" Of course, my answers were meant to be benign and as unrevealing as possible. So I said things like, "I worked out and made dinner," or "Nothing really, watched a movie on TV." I wanted him to participate in the give and take of conversation by asking me questions, too, but I didn't really want to give that much back. At any rate, I was thrilled that his conversational ability and turn taking were improving, and noted it in the chart.

On one of these Monday sessions, I asked Mark what he had done over the weekend. He told me, as I read the entry in his memory book, that he and his family had gone to church (they had attended chapel in the hospital). I asked Mark if he and his family usually went to church together. He said yes, and then said he'd like to ask me a question. I was thrilled that he would initiate this conversational skill, and enthusiastically replied, "Please, go ahead." He said, "Do you believe in God?"

I flinched. Here was a question that I was unlikely to discuss with many of my friends, and I certainly did not intend to discuss such an intimate issue with a brain-injured patient. On the other hand, wasn't I trying to help this patient be better able to engage in real, appropriate conversation? If that was the goal, didn't he deserve a real, conversational answer?

To this serious question, I thought, I had better give a serious answer. I should not be trite, and say something like "Well, of course," and smile, quickly adding "Now, let's get back to work." This patient was brain-injured, but he was more and more attuned to the emotional responses of others. I suppose I have got to answer this one honestly, I thought.

And so I said, "Well, I'm not sure." As I said these words, I commended myself for being honest, for treating this patient with respect enough to answer seriously. I was in no way prepared for his reaction. Mark's immediate response was, "What! You're supposed to be helping me, and you don't even believe in God!"

My heart and stomach both sank, and I realized that I had made a very grave mistake. After all these weeks of establishing a productive therapeutic relationship with Mark, I had perhaps blown it, irreparably, in one fell swoop. Here was a situation no one had talked to me about in any of my training, and one that I may or may not be able to figure my way out of.

"We can still work together on your memory and thinking skills, and it probably doesn't matter what I believe," I hastily explained, hoping for damage control. "Doesn't matter! How can it not matter?" Mark retorted. At last I resorted to, "Well, let's move on to some of our work today." As I wheeled him out of my office and down the hall to his next appointment, I was hoping that his anterograde amnesia would extend to this little episode, and not prevent us from working together productively through the end of his rehab.

Mark continued to make steady progress, and worked with me very cooperatively every day until his discharge to a community reentry program. He was enthusiastic about his move to the program, and his family was very happy. On his last day on our service, he and his wife thanked me for having worked with him, and I wished them all the best. I don't know if Mark remembered that conversation or not. We never spoke of that conversation or any related topic again. Because his memory had been slowly improving, it was very difficult for me to judge whether he might have remembered anything of what was to me a very eventful session. I always imagined that the rapport that Mark and I had during our therapy sessions was different after that day—not as easy, more work-related, fewer jokes and laughs, but always civil. This change in the therapeutic tone may have been all because of me. I felt uncomfortable. I felt that I had failed this patient, who had trusted me to at least appear to be everything that he needed me to be. He needed a therapist who believed in God, because he was depending on God to act through all of us for his recovery. Considering all of the whitewash jobs I usually did when asked about my weekend or other personal activities by patients, it wouldn't have hurt me to not really answer the brutal truth to this one, ultimately important, question.

A more experienced clinician would have seen this coming, I suppose. But I wasn't a more experienced clinician until I had this, and other, experiences. Long after Mark had been discharged, and I had seen many more patients of all different types, I became able to think about the strange relationships that therapists have with themselves when they are on the job. A good therapist needs to match styles with each individual patient. This does not just pertain to conversational tempo or topic, but to try to identify the perceived role that you are playing for that client. Some of it will be impossible or inappropriate for the therapist to try to fill, but some of it will really be the essence of what is important.

If Mark had not responded in this way to me, making me feel like a miserable failure for some short period of time, I might not have begun to think about the deeper roles that a speech pathologist is filling in a therapeutic relationship. I might have only kept thinking about my conversational style, my sentence length, my speech rate, and my facial expression. I might have kept business separate from personal existence. I might have thought that as a therapist I could get away with not being emotionally involved. Had I not exposed myself honestly, in that one utterance, and gotten a true response back from the patient, I might never have stopped to consider what the true meaning of a therapeutic relationship is.

Reflections

Revealing personal information to clients can be perceived in two different ways. Some consider self-disclosure a breach of professional boundary. Others view personal revelations as rapport building. The difficulty in clinical practice is that some disclosures may be boundary infractions, and others may serve the purpose of building a working relationship between a clinician and a client. This story describes one clinical scene early in my clinical fellowship during which I struggled to find an appropriate position between those dichotomies.

Self-disclosure has been investigated among physician-patient discourse (Beach et al., 2004). Categories of self-disclosure were identified from a set of 1,265 office visits that had been audio-recorded and transcribed. The authors reported that physician self-disclosure occurred in approximately 15% of all routine office visits. Self-disclosures were categorized as reassurance ("I've taken that, too"), counseling statements ("I've had my flu shot already"), rapport building ("I'd be nervous, too"), casual disclosures that had little to do with the patient, intimate disclosures ("I cried a lot when I got a divorce, too"), and extended narratives that went on at length but did not seem to be related to the patient's issues. Except for casual disclosures and extended narratives, it appeared that self-disclosing comments by the physician were made in an effort to foster reciprocity and trust that might also lead to compliance and cooperation. Clinician disclosure may produce more favorable perceptions in the patient, including liking the clinician more and finding the clinician more credible in regards to recommendations (Frank, Breyan, & Elon, 2000; Barrett & Berman, 2001).

In practice, it is informally reported that clients often reveal more of themselves to speech-language pathologists than to other allied health practitioners with whom they are working. We assume this is because we are the "talking" therapy, where conversation and getting one's ideas across is the central goal. Do we foster this? How so? Is our discourse in clinical sessions, particularly our self-disclosure, different from the disclosure of other kinds of allied health professionals, like occupational therapists or physical therapists? How do we talk about professional boundaries to our students and to each other?

Lunch Hour

"Hey," I said as I plopped into the chair. "How's your morning going?"

"OK," Susan said, rubbing her eyes.

"That patient I'm covering for Sharon is a real doozie—have you seen her?"

"No, but I heard Sharon say something about her last week. Got the impression she was a tough case."

"Yeah, nearly got a black eye in there this morning."

"Really, what happened? What is she, a traumatic brain injury? Car accident?"

"Yeah, I think it was one of those mangled up things that took hours for them to extricate her from the vehicle. Anyway, she's like 4 months post-accident already."

"So what happened?"

"The door's closed. I knocked, the sitter yells out to come on in. I open the door, the patient is lying on the bed, sitter's in the chair reading a book. I go up to the bedside, the patient is lying there, I introduce myself, say 'I'm Jackie and I'm your speech pathologist today. Do you remember Sharon? She came to see you last week.' The whole time the patient has been lying perfectly still, all of a sudden she grabs the table near her bedside, and screams 'I don't want any speech! I don't want any speech! Get the [bleep] out of here!'"

"Oh, my god." Susan is munching her salad.

I pause to get a bite of my yogurt. " 'Stacey, we're just going to talk,' I say, 'just have a conversation.' Apparently she didn't want to have any '[bleeping] conversation,' picks up the emesis basin off the table, and throws it at my head."

"Did she get you?" Susan is starting to snicker.

"No, she missed, and the basin was empty, which was a plus. It wasn't really that funny at the time, you know. I told her that it would be more appropriate to just ask me politely to leave."

Susan is laughing now through bites. "Did that work?"

"Not exactly. She started throwing every damn thing on the table, a fork, a teddy bear, her cards. The whole time, the sitter just stays in the corner reading his book."

"God, I don't remember Sharon saying anything about this patient throwing stuff."

"Maybe she likes Sharon better than she likes me."

"Who knows." Susan paused. "You just never think when you become a speech pathologist that you're going to be dodging emesis basins in the doorway."

"No kidding. Hey, do you remember that patient Bobby who was here for like 6 months? The one with the jargon aphasia? You know, he kept saying 'prable' for all of his nouns and verbs for the longest time?"

"Oh yeah, I remember him, he did really well by the time he was discharged. When was that, last year?"

"Yeah, almost a year and a half ago now. Well, I saw him and his mother this weekend. She called me and invited me over, saying that Bobby wanted to see me to thank me."

"Wow, that's nice. That practically never happens."

"I know, they are very nice people. When I got there, he and his mom are waiting for me, and he tells me everything that's been happening to him since his car accident, shows me his apartment, tells me his daily routine. He's doing pretty well now, living independently, working at a part-time job doing some low-level data entry or something, goes to a support group."

"Wasn't he the patient who had an accident on his way to his first day at his first job after college? Was he in engineering or chemistry or something?"

"Yeah, chemical engineering, had everything going for him, his fiancée left him after his car accident, his whole life now is completely screwed up compared to what he and his family anticipated."

"But he's doing much better than anyone expected him to at the beginning of his rehab, and he has you to thank for that. No one figured he'd be out living on his own. You were a good match for him as a therapist. And he knows it, that's why he wanted to see you."

"I suppose. Luck of the draw. He could have had you or any one of us, and he would have done as well."

"Don't be so sure. Sometimes you just get the right patient and you just get in the groove together, somehow it fits, and it makes a difference."

"That's true. It's like Stacey. I don't think she's ever thrown anything at Sharon, but I guess she just can't stand the look of me."

"So are you going to see her tomorrow? Or just monitor until Sharon comes back?"

"Oh, I guess I'll try it again tomorrow. But if she throws something at me for 2 or 3 days in a row, I might give up. We'll see."

"You never know, maybe she's going to do well like Bobby, in the end."

"Maybe." I heaved a sigh. Took the last bite of yogurt. "Yeah, now that I think about it, Bobby was pretty gorked out at about 4 months post, too. Who are you covering for Sharon?"

"I've got the sweetest little old white-haired lady with a right hemisphere stroke, and when I go in she doesn't stop talking until I leave! She goes, 'Oh dear, you have the cutest little dress on, and I love those shoes with it. I once had an outfit a lot like that, it was in 1943, right before the war . . .'"

"It's all reminiscence stuff?"

"She talks about everything, you know, typical right hemisphere disorder patient, she's tangential, verbose, but she's the cutest little old lady."

"How come I got the one who throws stuff? How come I didn't get the cute little old lady?"

"I'd guess you'd say it's the luck of the draw." Susan smiled.

Reflections

Attempts to find relationships between personality, as measured by a standard psychological test like the Minnesota Multiphasic Personality Inventory (MMPI), and general clinical effectiveness have been unsuccessful (Crane & Cooper, 1983). Personality matches between clinician and client, and perceived empathy in a clinician, do seem to relate to cooperativeness and compliance. The art of clinical practice is to attend closely enough to each client so that the clinician can make a reasonable estimate at what that client will respond to best. The clinician also develops a repertoire of demeanors and responses that are varied, like speech styles, in an attempt to foster reciprocity with the client and meet the client's needs. Narratives about how clinicians talk about this process, or about how and under what circumstances there was either a match or a mismatch between client and clinician, can help us to explore this part of our practice.

9

Overheard on the Bus

I climb the steps into the cool bus, air conditioning cranked just
high enough to make a stark contrast with the heat outside but not
enough to turn the bus into a moving icebox. I'm the first one in
and my favorite seat is available—passenger side, second row, next
to the window. I put my bag down on the aisle seat next to me.
I love this bus ride across the bay bridge in a cruising style bus with
high-back, plush seats that recline and tinted windows.

I nod to the white-haired lady who sits down in the front row.
I've seen her before on this bus; I think she works downtown.

Next comes a young black man with dreadlocks done up in a
scarf. A woman with a plain face, baseball hat, and a ponytail calls
down from the sidewalk, "Let me know when it's the last few seconds, I want to finish my coffee!"

The driver yells down, "Right now!" She's the youngest female
driver I've seen on this route.

The woman with the coffee cup in her hand ascends to the
fare collecting machine and starts to dig through the pockets of her
pants for change.

"You have a lid for that coffee?" the driver asks.

"No, but I seen people bring coffee on without lids all the time!"

"I wouldn't mind if you had a lid," the driver says, pulling out
a schedule or form of some kind and turning her head and attention away from the woman with a full cup of coffee.

"I walked all the way to Burger King to get change and just bought this coffee. Now I don't even have a chance to drink it?"

"Like I said, I wouldn't mind if you had a lid."

The man with dreadlocks jumps out of his seat and starts wandering around the bus. "You got an empty can of coke back here in this seat, and wrappers and stuff. They always got cokes and food back here."

"Well, you have to have a lid for the coffee."

The woman backs up, and dumps her nearly full cup of coffee in the nearby trash can. "I can't believe I can't have my coffee, when you got people eating whole meals on this bus." She gives the driver a look and takes a seat behind me.

A tall, slender young man looks up to the driver with his bus pass in his hand. He is wearing headphones and pulling a backpack on wheels behind him. He keeps his eyes straight on the fare machine, where he inserts his pass and waits for it to be spit back out at him. He grabs it and sits down quickly on the seat I've always seen him on. He rocks gently back and forth, listening to his music.

The driver looks around, no one else to board the bus. She closes the doors and we head off. "I had one woman," she says loudly enough for someone to hear, but to no one in particular, "sat right here next to me in the first row. Soon as we got started she broke her breakfast out right in front of me. I said, 'Ma'am, don't you see the sign NO FOOD NO DRINKS?' She just broke her breakfast right out, right in front of me!"

The bus is silent for an intersection or two. Then the man with dreadlocks calls out, "Did anyone see the presidential debates last night? Debate, debate, war and peace, they don't know nothing either one what they're doing!" No one on the bus responds.

"They keep fighting in Iraq, what about no food, no jobs right here? I got friends they be living in the streets. Nobody talking about them."

"Then you got some folks, they eat their whole meals right here on this bus!"

"OK, OK now," says the driver to the man.

The driver is paying close attention now as she negotiates narrow two-lane roads and turns. The next right-hand turn ahead is going to be a close call. She slowly inches the bus forward, gently turning to the right, watching the mirrors to avoid hitting the telephone pole on the corner.

"Look at this woman, she's got her car all the way over the line, and I'm here inching and sweating to make this turn. These people all the time over the line."

She completes the turn and we pull in the shopping mall for the next required stop. Only two or three people are waiting at the bus stop at this hour of the morning, and when our bus pulls up to the shelter, only one person makes any move to board.

"I'm moving slow, I'm moving slow." He looks young to me, maybe in his 30s or 40s, softened but muscular arms and shoulders draped with a tank top. A baseball hat and shorts complete the outfit, and he is carrying something in a tan plastic grocery bag.

He plunks down in the seat behind the woman who had lost her coffee, across the aisle from the man with dreadlocks.

"You're moving slow, we all moving slow my man," replies his new row-mate.

Our driver circles the bus out of the shopping mall, and returns to the main road by way of the same narrow right-hand turn we took to get in. She begins the turn, then stops the bus, dangling out in the intersection. She lays her hand on the horn and waits for a minute. When she releases her hand from the horn, she says, "Look at this one, over the line again. All day these people are over the white line. I'm making this turn to go in the mall and out, and everyone's over the line all day. Why should I be inching and working to get this bus around, when they so far over the line?"

The intimidated driver of a medium-sized sedan backs the car up as best he can. No doubt he would comply even faster if he could hear the accompanying remarks of the bus driver.

"You see that, we all be moving slow this morning!" comments the man with the dreadlocks.

"Yeah, I had a car accident," says the slow-moving man.

"You had a car accident!" echoes his row-mate.

"I got hit by a car."

"You got hit by a car! You doing well! When was this, 3, 4, 5 years ago?"

"I got hit by a car in August."

"August what year?"

"This year, 35 days ago!"

"This year, just last month?"

"Yeah, that's why I'm moving slow."

"You are doing very well, you got hit by a car last month. What were you, crossing the street?"

"I was on my bike."

"You were on your bike? Crossing illegally?"

"No, at the intersection. Ran a red light."

"The car ran a red light? Was he charged?"

"Yeah."

"With what, homicide? Attempted homicide?"

"No, charged with running a red light."

"That all? Does he have any money? You going to sue?"

"No, no money. I don't even know what is going to happen to him."

"That a shame, no money, when he ran a red light and hit you."

"Yeah, now I'm moving slow."

"How's your vision?"

There is a sudden pause in the quick exchange conversation, and I can't help but look behind just in time to get a glimpse of the slow-moving man place his artificial eye back in its socket.

"Whoa, that no good. And you telling me that this guy didn't have any money? Can you see all right?"

"That was from before, from Vietnam."

"Oh, that's not from your car accident?"

"No, long time ago."

"I knew a guy, walked across the street, got hit by a car, lost his vision. He sued because he couldn't work no more. That's why I wondered how's your vision."

"I'm doing all right now, I was in the hospital a few days, now I'm just moving slow. Can't drive."

"Well you are doing well my friend."

I'm thinking to myself, maybe a head injury in addition to losing his eye in Vietnam, maybe *another* head injury when he got hit by a car. I imagine he repeats this story to just about anyone who will listen for a second. I think back to a couple of other times when, waiting for a bus, a stranger has begun to tell me about his brain surgery, or his head injury. It seems that in the case of some "silent" disabilities, the affected person tells everyone he can about the problems that otherwise would not be casually observed— no canes, no wheelchairs, no braces.

"I gotta get off here." He gathers his grocery bag and pushes himself up against the seat arms.

"Hey, we got a gentleman here who needs to get off at this stop!" cries Dreadlocks.

"OK, OK," says the driver.

The bus comes to a stop. The driver signals for the person wanting to board to wait to give the slow-moving man enough time to get out. He steadily makes his way forward and down the steps, out the door.

A young man who looks like a student with a notebook decorated with blue ink doodles takes a seat next to the young man with head phones. He opens a catalog and starts paging through.

The bus heads out again into the busy main road. Looking around, I see that Headphones is staring at the pages of the catalog, which are covered with colorful electric guitars of all shapes and varieties. "You gonna buy a guitar?" he asks the new guy.

"Well, I'd like to but I have to save up some money."

"That one is like what the Beatles have. You know the Beatles, George Harrison?"

"Sure, but I think they had a different kind." He turns the page.

"The Beatles had one like this," Headphones says, pointing to a different one.

"Do you have a guitar?"

"No. I'm autistic."

"Oh, OK."

I am thinking, "Suspected diagnosis confirmed!" But much more than that, I marvel at this young man. Someone has taught him to take the bus himself every day and do something productive. He has developed a strategy for dealing with his disability. And I realize that, although I have seen him on the bus before, he has never forgotten his backpack or walkman or other items.

More pages get turned and Headphones keeps his eyes on the catalog.

"I'm sure you could teach me to play the guitar. Play the guitar like the Beatles," Headphones says.

"You like the Beatles?"

"Yeah, you can get all the Beatles records, like the old kind they still have them at stores and you can buy the old Beatles records."

"I like the Beatles, too."

I see ahead a school and just then the boy with the notebook twists, rings the bell, and jumps up to get off the bus.

Headphones follows him out the bus. I wonder if they had ever met before. I can't decide. I think that the young man with the catalog was tolerant and accepting. It makes me wonder if he has had experience with this young man before, or with autism, or some similar condition before. What a shame to assume that a tolerant person must have special experience that explains their patience and positivity!

We are nearing the end of the line and everyone else gets off at the next stop. As she walks by the driver, the woman with the ponytail says, "Say, I'm sorry I was rude about the coffee. I just wanted my coffee, it was a bad morning already."

"That's all right, don't worry about it," says the driver.

Dreadlocks moves up to the first row nearest the driver. I realize he and I are the only two remaining riders.

"Hey that was a hard story, this guy got hit by a car last month after losing his eye in Vietnam! That's a hard story."

"Yeah," responds the bus driver.

"I'm getting off at the next one."

"Right here?"

"Yeah. OK, see you."

"Yeah."

I say nothing as we get to the end of the line. I pick up my bag. "Thank you!" I say, as I walk down the stairs, leaving an empty bus.

Reflections

There's the short version and the long version of the story that sums us up to others. On this day on the bus, I came across two short stories that I was professionally familiar with—"I was hit by a car" and "I'm autistic." I know, probably in much greater detail than my two fellow riders with these stories, the science underlying the nature of these disorders and their treatment. But I don't know what it is like to feel a need to explain to strangers why something I'm doing is different. The gentleman who'd had a car accident was "moving slow," and then told his story to his chatty row-mate. The young man who announced "I'm autistic" was maybe trying to explain his magnetic focus on the catalog pictures of the guitars, and his slight rocking back and forth on the bus seat.

Sometimes we run into clients in the community long after we have worked with them. Chance meetings of that kind present their own interactional challenges; either the client or the clinician might be embarrassed, overjoyed, or neutral about seeing each other. Reactions may not match; the client may be embarrassed and the clinician happy, or vice versa. In this story, I was in the position of overhearing individuals with communication disorders handle their disability in a public setting without having any previous knowledge of those individuals. How do our clients manage the mundane details of living with their disability? How many times during the day do they find themselves explaining, or avoiding, being embarrassed, or taking a devil-may-care attitude?

We know relatively little about the ultimate or long-term outcomes of our clients. Some clinicians have the luxury of working in settings in which they have the opportunity to follow up with clients years later, but many clinicians do not work in the circumstances that allow them to do so. We need to rely on our clinical literature to describe what clients with various disorders can or might do several years after intervention. This is particularly true when we are working with clients who have chronic disabilities, such as adults with neurogenic impairments or children with language disorders (Fujiki & Brinton, 2005).

10

The Optimist and the Fatalist

"It may be hard to believe now," Herb says in his booming, authoritative, and enthusiastic voice, "but when I first woke up after my stroke I could say"—he pauses for dramatic effect—"nothing! Not one word!"

I had invited Herb to talk at a meeting for students, faculty and clients, and other community members. He was visiting Tampa and I was thrilled to see him again and have him talk on campus.

I hadn't seen Herb for about a year, since the last National Aphasia Association conference. At that meeting he had captured the attention of the audience of 300 people living with aphasia, their families and friends, and the professionals who strive to help them. I knew from conversation with Herb that he had been through big personal changes during the course of that year, including a divorce and a move to live in a different city. But in the face of sadness, disappointment, and stressful challenges he had maintained his contagious optimism.

"I remember, during my first few days in the hospital," Herb continued to his small audience in our classroom, "the doctor standing at my bedside. He pulled a pen out of his pocket, and said to me, 'What is this called?' I struggled. I knew I knew the name of that thing.

I set my lips, and triumphantly blurted out 'Pen!' The doctor showed me his watch, and asked me what it was called. Again I yelled out 'Pen!' The third time, the doctor picked up a cup from my bedside tray, and I called out 'Pen!' For days I said nothing but 'Pen!'

"A couple of weeks later, I was watching the Super Bowl with my mother and brother. It occurred to me that what would be great would be a pizza. So I called out, 'Pen!' My mother said, 'What, I don't understand what you mean!' I called out again, 'Pen!' My mother again tried, 'Do you need to go to the bathroom?'

"With a great effort, I thought of how a pizza would smell and taste. This was one of my favorite things—especially coming from Chicago. So, putting all my energy behind it, I yelled out, 'I want a pizza!' These were the first words I had said other than 'pen' in weeks! Unfortunately, I was so tired by the time the pizza was delivered that I slept right through it!"

Herb's planned laugh line was cheerfully received and the audience giggled. Herb presented the tragedy of his loss in a way that was palatable and allowed the audience to imagine itself in that situation. His soft-shoe approach contrasted with the way some people talked about their stroke. Painting it in harsh, dramatic tones tended to make listeners mentally distance themselves from such grief and pain.

Although I had heard Herb talk in similar situations before, I was drawn in by the telling of his story. If, at 27 years of age, I had awoken in a hospital bed to only be able to say the word "pen," would I ever be able to make an amusing story out of it? For that matter, had there been any difficulties in my past about which I could now make a pleasant story?

"So then, after my first couple of days of speech therapy, I could say 'I want a . . . pizza!' Herb continued. "My family even brought me a pizza, but really all I wanted was a straw in my water!" I look around the audience and see smiles and hear chuckles.

What about my own divorce, I mused. How do I usually tell that story? Yes, I've got it boiled down to a short version that I can tell, and I can elaborate on details to a sympathetic girlfriend, but I don't recall ever telling the story in what might be considered an amusing way. It's not that I take it overly seriously, but even being happily remarried hasn't quite shown me the funny side of the old divorce story.

No, I think, I am much more likely to tell the story with an ending that goes something like, "Well, I guess it's not too surprising that I made a bad choice the first time around." And that moral of the story comes with detailed rationale, too, if the talk and wine are flowing between friends.

"After about a year," Herb says, "I was discharged from speech therapy because I could say when I was hungry, or thirsty, or what I needed basically. But I was young; I expected to go back to work. So I set out to find a job. After the first 20 interviews that didn't go so well, I decided that my first job was to get a job. So for a year I sent out resumes and went to over 100 job interviews." Here the audience intakes a great breath. "For each interview, I practiced before I went and analyzed what went wrong afterwards. I decided that, with practice, I would get better and better at doing job interviews, and when I got good enough at it, I would get a job. And eventually I did get a job, at the blood bank." The room filled with spontaneous applause of his victory.

Have I ever persisted at anything for so long? Could I ever persist at anything for so long? Persistence in a degree program isn't anything like what Herb has done. To persist in a degree program, even to get through graduate school, I periodically succeeded—each assignment of each course passed. How long could I persist if each time I turned in my work, I failed? How many degree programs would I have been willing to apply to, if I at first had been rejected? Would I have persisted through over 100 applications or interviews for anything, ever? Herb's story was one of persistence and ultimate triumph. I realize that I would have told myself a story of persistent failure with the title "Jackie fails to get a job again." Byline: "I'm sure I won't get the next one, either."

Herb is telling us that he attributes his achievements to his positive attitude. He is assuring all of us that we can accomplish our goals, too, with belief and a smile. I think of all the different days over the years that I have spoken to Herb. If he has had self-doubts, he has kept them to himself. I think of him smiling and saying, "Try, try again!"

I know I have never arrived at maintaining such a consistently positive outlook, even for my "public" face, under much less trying circumstances. In order to get through things, I consider the worst possible outcome and convince myself that it is not really that bad.

Swimming in an outdoor pool and hearing thunder, I once rationalized that being struck by a lightning in the university pool would very likely be the only way my death could hit the newspaper—"Faculty Member Killed by Lightning in University Pool"—and my surviving spouse would probably be eligible for some extra money. Sailing offshore in a small boat, I don't think confidently that we are skilled enough and have the right equipment to stay safe. Rather, I think that being lost at sea is a much more interesting way to go and will make a better story than other more usual end-of-life alternatives. This way of thinking is not classically considered a "positive outlook."

I reflect on a book I recently read, in which the author (Norton, 1989) asks people to fill in the following blank: "Life is like _____." He describes attitudes that are observed in these stories as being either positive or negative, and either passive or more active. The combination of negative and passive is termed *fatalist*, while negative-active is called *antagonist*. The combination of positive with passive is *spectator*, and positive-active is *enthusiast*. There's no question where Herb's approach lies along these dimensions—an unabashed enthusiast. I plot my own attitude more towards the negative, and although I am loath to describe myself as an antagonist—it sounds so mean!—I doubt I could be considered passive.

So, if I could only say the word *pizza*, would I think to myself "I'll never be able to say anything but 'pizza'"? Could I think that and still persist in practicing every day? Could I become more positive if I needed to? Would I?

Herb is ending his talk exactly on time, as he promised he would when he first started. I rarely time my talks so well. He appears to feel he has done well, accepts the many compliments gracefully and sincerely. I always feel that I have done poorly, and in my heart rarely accept a compliment, although I have learned to be polite.

If I had a stroke like Herb, would I achieve so much? Could I achieve so much? The nagging doubt that I couldn't or wouldn't and the admiration that Herb has done so is all wrapped into the hug I give him when all the questions are asked and the hearty applause has ended.

Reflections

The gentleman in this story is really named Herb Silverman, and he has given me his full permission to include this story about him and to use his real name. I sent a draft of this story to Herb, and he responded by sending me back his version of how he went from saying "pen" to "I want a pizza!" I have incorporated his version of the story here.

In response to reading this story, Herb wrote the following to me:

> I read your chapter three times and each time I was very moved by what you said. The fact that I was a positive impact not only for the people in your story, but you, yourself, is very satisfying to me. . . . Considering we have been friends for 16 years and all of the changes that I believe both of us have done, sometimes it all comes together like a big quilt. Some of the pieces are not in place yet, some of the pieces are finished, some of the pieces are tattered and need to be repaired, but we still keep working at it.

Our attempts at reciprocity in the clinical relationship don't often extend to letting our clients know what they have done for us, or how they have made us feel, or what they have taught us. I acknowledge that it is the rare set of working and clinical circumstances that might allow us to share in such a way with our clients comfortably. In the case of Herb and me, we stayed in touch and have known each other long enough to share these thoughts with each other. I suspect, though, that there are more opportunities to let clients know what they have done for us than we take advantage of.

11

Bitter Memories

I hang up the phone, shaken. A knock at the door comes so quickly that I don't have time to compose myself.

"I know you're in there," Kathy calls amiably.

I reach over and pull open the door, standing well in the office. Kathy has worked with me for several years, and knows my stance means she should walk in. She moves in close in front of me, shutting the door behind her.

"What's up?" she asks gently.

"I got a call from Mrs. Josephson; you remember her husband, Joe?"

"How could I forget Joe Josephson? He was adorable. He smiled all the time. He could say his first name but never reliably his last name, so he just said 'Jo-Jo.'"

"Yeah, that's him. I was so excited to hear from Mrs. 'Jo-Jo'; it's been, what, about a year since he was here in the clinic?"

"Yeah, that's about right."

I pause. I swallow. How can I retell something so painful, so horrifying to my dear friend and colleague? Kathy comes off as a toughie but can easily come to tears over truly sad events.

She looks at me, silent and waiting.

I swallow again. "Jo-Jo committed suicide about a month ago. Mrs. Josephson wanted to call and let us know, and ask us to take her off our newsletter mailing list. It's too hard for her to keep getting our mailings, now."

"Oh, my god." Kathy takes in breath. She is trying not to cry.

"I know. Sit down." I guide her to an empty chair.

We sit in silence for a minute.

"What happened?" Kathy asks, grabbing a Kleenex from the box on my desk.

How can I retell the details that Mrs. Josephson told me? The image is too awful for me. I don't have the courage to conjure up such an image in any one else's mind.

"He, uh, committed suicide. He was afraid that his aphasia was getting worse, and he was starting to have trouble driving, and he was worried that he would become a burden to his family."

"Jesus! How could he think that! He'd been doing so well. Wasn't he still doing his volunteer job that we set up for him?"

"Yes, apparently he was, but he thought he was having trouble driving. And when he tried to take the bus one day, he got lost and confused and missed his whole shift. Mrs. Josephson said he was so mortified it was everything she could do to get him to go back to it. When he did, he cut his time down to only 2 days a week without telling her. She didn't even know about the schedule cut until after he died, when the people from the hospital volunteer service came to the memorial service."

"I can't believe it."

"I know." Tears are filling my eyes now.

"What—how did he do it?" she asks, timidly. Maybe she doesn't want to know, maybe she really doesn't, I think.

I replay Mrs. Josephson's voice on the phone in my mind. She was so matter-of-fact, reporting, perhaps her best defense now. She told me how Jo-Jo had given her no warning signs that she could tell. He seemed his cheerful self. But one night while she was soundly sleeping, he drove the car to the Sunshine Skyway Bridge, the "Golden Gate Bridge" of Florida. He left the car parked neatly in the trouble lane with a full tank of gas—Mrs. Josephson said he never liked her to be low, he always kept the tank filled up for her. Somehow in the cold, dark night he crawled and climbed his way over the railings and the structures, without the use of his hemiparetic right hand, found a spot to slide through, and jumped 175 feet to the blackness below. His mangled, bloated body was found floating by an early morning fisherman after he had been missing for 48 hours.

My memory of Jo-Jo is of an eternally cheerful and helpful person. He was always alert to others, lending whatever help he could, if only a pat on the back. Often, walking past me in the clinic hallway, he had patted my shoulder and given me a smile and a thumbs-up. I always felt something must be going right when Jo-Jo cheered me on.

I cannot combine my memory of happy Jo-Jo and the awful picture of him planning and carrying out such a desperate act. I don't want to think about Jo-Jo, cold, climbing and finding his way out to the edge of the bridge. I can't stomach the thought of him filling the gas tank for the last time. The images are swirling around in my mind's eye, making me dizzy and sick.

Kathy is still looking at me. "I said, how did he do it?"

"I just can't tell you."

"Why?"

"Because it's too awful for me to think about, I can't say it out loud, and I don't see why anyone else should be burdened with it."

"That bad?" she said, blowing her nose.

"Yes. I'll go around to the rest of the staff after therapy is over with today and let people know."

"Want some help?"

"No, it's all right; I get paid the big manager bucks for doing the dirty work." I make a reference to our ongoing joke about my small but supposedly meaningful "administrative supplement."

"Kathy, why don't you leave early today? Just go home now. I'll let the others know and close up shop today." I give my assistant what I am wishing for.

"Are you sure?" she asks.

"Yes, I'm sure."

I am lecturing on psychosocial issues in aphasia in a graduate course. My standard set of slides includes a discussion of depression and also suicide. My lecture notes include basic statistics and appropriate courses of action for the speech-language pathologist in the event that a client makes comments that could be suicidal. During the lecture, I try to listen to myself.

"I've known of former clients of mine who, long after they were discharged from therapy, committed suicide. I believe that speech-language pathologists don't often know when this happens or how frequently it does happen, because we don't usually get to follow our clients for years after they've been in therapy. But it does happen, it can happen, and we need to be alert to signs of suicide and take appropriate action."

My mind flashes on Jo-Jo. Could we have told him something, or told him something more frequently, that might have changed anything? Could we have done a better job of ensuring he understood that his aphasia was not progressive? Did we place too much emphasis on his volunteer job, thus leading him to wrap his whole post-stroke identity around his ability to get to that job and do it? No way to know.

I have never told anyone about how Jo-Jo died. I have never been able to bring the words to my mouth. I hear Mrs. Josephson's voice on the phone clearly, even now, 10 years later, but I can't say any of those same words aloud.

I look up and realize that my students are all looking at me wondering if I'm OK after such an extended pause in the lecture and discussion.

"I've known clients who a year after discharge committed suicide," I repeat. "So that's why I think it's important to think about this for any client, not just your clients with aphasia."

I end the lecture with stories of people I've known who live successfully with aphasia. I try to rinse the bad taste out of my mouth with a sweet one.

After class, one of my most conscientious students waits to talk to me after everyone else has left the room. I don't know Margaret very well but I like her.

"Dr. Hinckley," she starts in her upright voice, "I want to thank you for bringing up the topic of suicide today in class. My cousin attempted suicide 5 years ago, and ever since then my whole family has been very active in suicide education and prevention. Few people talk about it and you're the first instructor I've had who raised it in class, and I just want to say I appreciate it."

"Thank you for the comment, Margaret. I'm sorry to hear about your cousin. Suicide is hard to talk about under every circumstance, it seems."

I haven't ever told the details of Jo-Jo's death to anyone. But 10 years later the image that his wife's description forged in my mind is still as clear as the moment I hung up the phone.

Reflections

Speech-language pathologists know that clients can be at risk for suicide, and the potential for suicide is sometimes discussed relative to the psychosocial aspects of living with any particular communication disorder. In my research, I could not find any publications that dealt in detail with suicide and communication disorders, except for general references about risk, signs, and basic suicide prevention.

Assuming that my experiences as a clinician are typical, each one of us has come to know about the suicide of a client at some point. I know of three of my former clients who committed suicide, long after they had been discharged from services. There are so many clients I have worked with about whom I know nothing after they left the caseload.

Clinical psychologists are by nature of their profession at greater risk of handling clients who ultimately commit suicide. Meichenbaum (2006) reports that one in six graduate students in clinical psychology will experience the suicide of a client, and that this rate does not diminish among practicing psychologists as experience increases. Among young people with TBI, a group that often experiences cognitive-communicative disorder and is served by speech-language pathologists, perhaps as many as 25% attempt suicide (Simpson & Tate, 2005). Those with post-injury histories of psychiatric/emotional disturbances and substance abuse were 21 times more likely to attempt suicide than TBI survivors without such post-injury histories.

What are the estimated rates for speech-language pathologists? Do we know how frequently it occurs? Relative to its occurrence, are we sufficiently educated about suicide prevention to be sensitive to signs that warrant referral? If we do know about a client who commits suicide, how do we handle it? Where can we tell the story? One purpose of clinical anecdotes is to handle perceived failures, and suicide is often experienced as a type of failure by clinicians (Meichenbaum, 2006). In my own case, I admit telling the story to myself as a way of working things out, but never really being able to share the details with anyone—not a colleague, not a friend. Until the day that I wrote this story, it was too sad for me to put into words.

12

A Group of Life Stories

"You have all been in aphasia group together before, isn't that right?" I ask.

The men gathered around the conference table nod.

"Not me," says Lou.

"Yes, but . . . " says Burt, waving his hand back and forth between Lou, himself, and the others.

"Well, yes, before," Lou says.

"You've all met before, but Lou hasn't been in a group with the rest of you before, is that right?" I ask.

Nods of agreement all around.

"What are we, what are we, what are we doing? Going to do?" asks Charlie, in his slow, overarticulated speech.

"What would you like to do?" I counter.

"You tell us!" smiles Burt.

I look around the table, and they all smile and nod.

"How about if I suggest a couple of things, if you like one of them, fine, if not, we'll all come up with a better idea. OK?"

"Well, you tell us," Charlie clarifies. His tone suggests that he is telling me how an aphasia group is supposed to go. As a substitute leading this particular group, I find myself a little hesitant to shake up the dynamics that they expect.

"Well, even though we've all met before, we may not know that much about each other." I look around the table. I had selected a seat along the side of the table, not at the head. I hadn't wanted anyone to think I was the leader—I had wanted to position myself as a member of the group. A round table would have been nice, but I didn't have it available.

"So," I continue, "one thing we might consider doing is to sketch out a story of our lives. Then we can share as much or as little with the rest of the group as we want."

I pause, choosing the words to present the second idea I was planning to propose.

"Good! Good idea!" pronounces Peter.

"Lets do that," agrees Tim.

A little surprised by their quick enthusiasm, I ask if they wouldn't like to hear my other idea.

"This one good," says Lou, the others chiming in with OKs.

"Great," I say, smiling.

I make sure there are plenty of paper and pencils and pens in front of each of them.

"Let's take a few minutes and consider the story of our lives. If you were telling your own story, how would it go? What are the most important events? What have been important values or themes in your lives? Let's each sketch, draw, or write a little summary of our lives. You can do it any way that you want. Do you each understand what I mean?"

Another round of yeses and OKs. This was my first session with this group and my impression was that, for a group of people with aphasia group experience, they were the most agreeable lot I'd ever run across.

We each begin to write. I took a few minutes because I hadn't quite considered how I might represent my own life story in some kind of sketch or diagram.

Burt looked across the table at me with my pen poised above the blank sheet. "You too?" he grinned.

"Yes, I'm doing it, too, and I have to think for a minute how I want to show things."

"Yes, yes," agreed Lou. "Thinking!"

A quiet lull of thinking settled on us all, heads bent down. I hear the clock ticking and the hum of the refrigerator in the corner.

"Education, education," says Burt, writing the letter *E* and looking around the table.

"Spelling it?" asks Jim.

"Yes, yes, education."

Tim writes it on a piece of scratch paper and it is passed down the side of the table to Burt, like butter at the dinner table.

Quiet overtakes us again. I try to glance subtly at my watch; the session needs to end on time so they can go to their next appointments.

Heads begin to rise, and we are looking around the table at each other.

"All set? Has everyone got started at least?" I ask.

More nodding.

"OK, I thought the next thing we might do is buddy up, and we can each tell one other person at the table some of the story of our lives. What events were most important, and why? OK?"

"Yes, so, me and time, and . . . " Peter gestures pairs around the table, and in so doing, gives us our buddy assignments.

We each turn to our buddy. Lou and I are seated next to each other; we swivel in our seats. He starts right in. Lou shows me a graph on which he has written words and partial words. A line is drawn, showing a gradual increase, a plateau at the highest point, a sudden drop to bottom again, and a slow rise up to what seemed like a halfway point.

Lou explains to me about his schooling, his years of military service, and his successful development of his own business. His store, his marriage, and his children he locates spatially on the high plateau of his graph. Pointing to the precipitous drop, he says simply "Stroke." Lou tells me that since the stroke he has only returned to 40% or 50% of his abilities.

As Lou is finishing, he looks around realizing that the sound of others talking simultaneously had ended and he was the only one speaking.

"Forty-fifty? You? Now? C'mon . . . " Bert says encouragingly.

"You're speaking very well," says Charlie.

"But, reading, writing—nothing," counters Lou.

"Comes in time, comes in time," adds Tim wisely.

"Me nothing before, now spelling, better and better," adds Peter.

"Well, thank you, but 50", concludes Lou, indicating that the encouragement had not changed his mind.

"And you now," Lou says, turning to me.

"OK, I will share mine with the group," I say.

I had drawn a timeline that curved the length of the paper in a large S-shape. I told the dates of my degrees and had written "WORK" in capitals over long stretches of time. At the end I had left a lot of blank timeline culminating in an arrow.

"No children?" asked Burt.

"No, no children," I answer.

I realize that I am uncomfortable with how sparse my life seems when asked to put it down in such a condensed form. It seems like a particularly simple and easy life compared to the complexities represented in my fellow group members' stories.

Each group member in turn ran down his list of educational and occupational achievements, noting marriages and births of children. Everyone but Tim included the stroke as a major event.

"Tim," I say, "I notice that you are the only one who did not include the stroke on his timeline. Did you do that on purpose?"

"Yes," he says.

I pause, hoping he'll elaborate.

"The stroke," Tim says, "I'm over it."

Laughter breaks out, relieving the tenseness of a quiet mood.

"Hey, we're over it!" repeat Burt and Peter, still laughing.

I look at my watch. Hard to imagine a better ending to the group session.

"Thank you all very much for sharing your life stories. I really enjoyed learning more about each one of you."

"Thank you," says Charlie. "A good session."

"Thank you," I say.

I watch them leave, relieved and satisfied to see each one smiling as he walks out the door.

Reflections

This single session was a condensed version of each group member's self-defining moments, including my own. It's not always easy to boil down one's life into a short list of major events. Doing so can be either pride-inspiring, disconcerting, or possibly both. If I had not done the activity with my clients, I might not have been sensitive to the gamut of their possible emotional reactions. The group members, including myself, were able to relate to each other by the items they selected to share about their life stories.

All but one of the members of the group identified the stroke as a critical, possibly self-defining, moment. Tim's victorious cry of "I'm over it!" seemed to be his way of saying that he was not interested in having the stroke define him or his life. It was readily taken up by two of the other group members, who seemed to immediately grasp the importance of being "over it."

13

My Clients, Myself

"She already knows she has it," I hear the doctor tell his residents and medical students about me through the thin examining room door. They are talking about the results of an eye examination they had completed on me through the morning. "So we don't have to worry about that." He sounds relieved that he will not have to break the news of the diagnosis on me.

He knocks two times quickly on the door and walks in without waiting for a response, followed by his entourage. He shakes my hand again, thanking me for my patience through the morning's tests. "You know you have retinitis pigmentosa, you've told us at the beginning that you were already aware of that." He is explaining himself to me or to his students, I don't know which.

"Yes, I've known about that for a long time now, since I was 16, as I explained before," I reply.

"So the preliminary results of the tests this morning confirm that. I don't know that we have that much new to tell you."

"Well, as I indicated this morning at the beginning of the appointment, my main interest in coming to your specialty clinic here was to get an idea of the prognosis."

"You understand that it is a progressive disorder—that means there is gradual deterioration of the retina over time."

"Yes, I understand what the disease is. But what I'd like to know is, based on my current status and the rate of progression so far, what can I expect in the future?"

"It is very difficult for us to tell people what will happen in the future. The disease affects everyone differently and progression can occur sometimes slowly and sometimes more rapidly."

"I understand that. I understand about individual differences. But I wonder if, based on your clinical experience, you could give me a general picture of what I might expect given my status so far."

"I really would rather not do that," the doctor replies with a slight curve of the lips, "because it might be wrong; you can't really count on what I might say as an absolute."

"I understand that. I'm a health professional, too, a speech-language pathologist, and I work up at the hospital. I understand that a prognosis is your best guess based on your experience of seeing other patients in similar circumstances. I won't hold you responsible or take your estimate for gospel."

"Thank you for telling me that you understand the idea of a prognosis. But that also means you know how hard it is to give one to somebody."

"Yes, I do," I reply, getting frustrated now, "but I'd like to make things clearer. Within the last year I completed my degree and now I'm working in a career. I need to know what I am going to do with my life. I need to have a basic guess, even if it turns out to be wrong, on which I can plan. Do I need to think about a different career? A different way to do my job? Or can I plan to do this job for a good while and then do something different later? I just need to know how to get on with things."

"I understand your dilemma," he replies, and I am not at all sure that he does. "Perhaps I could refer you to our social worker. She is very good."

"Well, I would be willing to talk to a social worker if she could help me think about resources and information that I need to figure out what to do with my life. But that is still going to be hard to do if you don't give me a general idea of a prognosis."

There is a pause and I'm still not sure this internationally known expert is going to give me the courtesy of his clinical knowledge. "Please, I'm begging you. I promise not to sue you. I'll sign a waiver, for goodness' sake. What do I have to do to persuade you that I am not going to break down in hysterics, pursue legal action, or ask you to sign a guarantee? I just want a normal part of the medical process, and that is a basic prognosis. I mean, really, how would you feel if you were sitting on my side of the examining room?"

He looks at me with saddened, sympathetic eyes as though he really could imagine what it might be like if our roles were reversed. "Yes, I do understand. Based on my experience with people who have your variant of the disease, and based on an estimated rate of progression according to your medical history, by the time you are 40 years old you can expect . . . " And he gives me a prognosis. He tells me what kinds of things I will be able to see and do in 15 or 20 years, by the time I am 40, and by the time I am 50 years old.

Now that those 15 or 20 years have passed, and I am halfway between those two age points, I am happy that I am better off than the prognosis he gave me that day. But the prognosis I got that day allowed me to reconsider myself: who I might be and how I might be functioning later down the road. Over the next few years after that prognosis, I visualized myself living differently than I was living then. After finishing graduate school, I had a rough outline in mind about the way my life and more specifically my career might go. That story needed to be revised, based on the information that my reluctant but expert doctor gave me that day. Like reading a mystery and guessing "whodunit," I had received significant new information and I needed to imagine an alternative ending.

Reflections

My doctor in this case did not mean to frustrate me, nor did he intend to do me any harm, and by the end of the interaction he gave me the information I was seeking and he did well by me. In my memory he is a kind, almost-too-sympathetic, well-intentioned clinician. My memory of him is positive, more than likely because he finally gave me the information I wanted. If he had not done so, or done so vaguely, I would have been very dissatisfied and unhappy.

My doctor and his staff at that particular clinic were used to diagnosing patients for the first time. They were experienced at delivering the news to people who had no idea what was going on with their vision. Their typical job was to show patients a new book, opening it to the first page, telling them something like "You haven't ever considered the possibility of having something wrong with your vision, but that is now the story that you are living in." I'm sure I was an exception. I had already started reading the book and was halfway through it before I even came in the door that morning. I wanted to get some clues about how the ending might go; I'd already been through the first chapter or two.

This personal event is a very meaningful one to me in regards to my clinical practice. Because of this personal experience, I have a strong opinion about being vague and waffling about prognoses. On the other hand, as speech-language pathologists we rarely have sufficient empirical evidence on which to make a data-based prognosis. Any prognosis is based solely on clinical experience. We do not want to be cruel, or stifle hope with any comment we would make. On the other hand, assuming some of our clients have personalities similar to mine, at least some of our clients want to have a rough idea so that future life planning can go on. Indeed, a recent review of the published narratives of adults living successfully with aphasia suggested that a common theme among narratives was the ability to look to the future and set new goals (Hinckley, 2006). Goal setting has been identified as a key ingredient to successful aging, as well (Riediger, Freund, & Baltes, 2005). It is only possible to set goals when we can imagine a narrative framework for the future.

How does a good clinician figure out what to say and how to say it when giving prognostic information? Maybe more stories about successes and failures will help us explore this issue.

Section IV

Using a Narrative Approach

14

The Development of the Clinical Self

OVERVIEW

The narratives we create with our clients in the clinical setting reveal important individual perspectives of our clients. A narrative-based approach also acknowledges the equal contribution of the clinician to the narrative. Therefore, clinician discourse during therapeutic encounters, as well as how clinicians talk with each other and to themselves, can help to reveal what is really happening in clinical practice. Finally, narratives are important formal and informal tools for training and continuing professional development in speech-language pathology.

LEARNING OBJECTIVES

At the end of this chapter, the reader will be able to:

1. Identify at least three aspects of clinician-client discourse that have been or could be studied within the context of speech-language pathology practice.

2. Describe the links between narrative and the development of empathy and reflection, including at least one specific method for facilitating the development of empathy in a training program.

3. Describe the potential roles of narrative in the handling of medical/clinical errors.

Narrative as a Tool to Develop Clinical Expertise

Identity can be seen as being constructed via a narrative process. Identity is important to our clients; hopefully what we are engaged in therapeutically with our clients will not detract from and will perhaps enhance our clients' views of themselves and what they will be able to accomplish in the future. Their self-narrative will have to accommodate newly developed abilities and habits. Narrative can be used as a mechanism to facilitate adaptation to illness, injury, or disability, lessening stress and decreasing feelings of isolation and alienation.

For the speech-language pathologist, narrative provides a window to our clients' experiences, and listening carefully to the metaphors and structures they use may allow us to more effectively and efficiently facilitate compliance and positive outcomes. Patient care is a result of a complex system of competing agendas between the clinician and the client (Aita, McIlwain, Backer, McVea, & Crabtree, 2005). Communication within the clinician-client encounter reveals the landscape of these motives and intentions, and can also reveal the resulting meaning that is co-constructed.

Narrative can and should be applied to more than just the client side of the therapeutic equation. The speech-language pathologist constructs his or her own self-narrative. The experienced clinician has also incorporated aspects of her own work culture into her own narrative perspective, and constructs a narrative about her own life as a clinician. Clients get under our skin, no matter how thick-skinned we believe ourselves to be. Our interactions with our clients become a part of our own narrative, just as we become part of our clients' narratives.

Narrative is an important way to learn and change behaviors. This can be applied to formal educational approaches in both pre-professional training and professional development. During patient and professional education, narratives are grounded in clinical experience. Narratives are more likely to be remembered than a statement of general principle. A listener projects him- or herself into a story, and thus more readily questions whether he or she would have acted the same way, or come to a similar conclusion. The listener becomes more cognitively engaged in a narrative, usually in a personalized way. Case-based learning and learning from the narratives of other professionals are two ways to incorporate a narrative approach into professional training.

Finally, the role of narratives in clinical research can help to generate new hypotheses by exploring difficult to quantify concepts and issues. The lived experience of the patient becomes a starting point for the generation of a research agenda, rather than identifying patient issues based on what a clinician imagines about patients' experiences. Similarly, the lived experience of a clinician could be an equal source of research interest; clinicians' emotional and psychological workings also contribute to the construction of meaning in the clinical process.

There are three broad areas in which narrative is an important tool in the development of the clinician. First, narrative is a powerful tool to incorporate into formal training programs to develop reflection and problem-solving skills. Second, narrative is one way to think about the clinical interaction—not just a single client contact but the whole journey taken by a client and clinician together. Finally, reflection and problem-solving skills are put to the test to confront and learn from errors. Narratives are ways in which we can learn to avoid practice errors and can process and cope with committed errors.

Narrative and the Clinical Interaction

Two clinicians with the same amount of experience administering the same treatment and therapy task could potentially produce different therapy outcomes because of the nature of the clinician-client relationship (Horton & Byng, 2000; Treadway, 2004). Several descriptive frameworks have been developed to classify the frequency and types of interactions between clinicians and clients. These frameworks generally result in descriptions of the interaction in terms of the frequency of responses in a priori designated categories. Even those researchers who are interested in investigating clinician-client interaction acknowledge that this is a relatively sterile way to consider the meaning that emerges from a therapeutic interaction. Narrative approaches have the potential to capture the story line of either the patient or the clinician or both as they form a therapeutic relationship. Conversation and discourse analysis can also help to reveal important patterns or differences that help to make the clinical relationship more or less productive.

Narrative between a Client and a Clinician

At the beginning of any clinical relationship, it is common for the speech-language pathologist to ask the client to talk about her communication concerns in some way. Speech-language pathologists are especially attuned to listening to their client's perspective. This not only aids the clinician in arriving at an appropriate communication diagnosis, but it identifies the client's personal and social communication concerns that may serve as areas in which to target intervention. The words that the client selects to describe her situation, the metaphors inherent in her talk, and the paralinguistic and nonlinguistic aspects of her discourse may all be revelatory.

Health professionals bring a certain schema into their clinical interactions, typically stemming from the medical culture and context. This point of view may not be the patient's perspective—at least not initially. An individual who is sick and wants to be well ascribes a high degree of power to the health professionals on which he or she must rely. Thus, the patient may take on elements of the narrative forms used by health professionals. This is not necessarily bad, as patients may need to integrate medical information into their everyday lives. For their part, health professionals might be more effective or efficient at conveying certain medical information or facilitating compliance with treatment regimens if the patient's narrative was given more serious attention. Integrating aspects of the patient's narrative more specifically into the practitioner's communications might produce desirable outcomes within the health encounter.

The use of medical terminology and medical language by the clinician in a health service encounter tends to lead the patient to develop a medically-based story about self and the illness (Eggly, 2002) The patient begins to use the same terminology experienced in the medical setting and therefore may develop a story for him- or herself in the role of the patient. If the clinician incorporates nonmedical or non-illness terminology into the clinical interaction, patients may more easily be able to integrate their perceptions of themselves apart from the illness with the health issue. This allows the patient to create a narrative that weaves language aspects of the story about herself prior to illness with her current health status. Thus, clinicians are encouraged to use nonmedical, subjective language in their clinical interactions in addition to using medical terminology to describe the patient's plight (Waxman, 2005).

The linguistic-cultural backgrounds of the patient and the clinician will affect the ability of the patient to explain herself to the clinician, and the ease with which the clinician-patient dyad co-constructs the story of the illness. Moss and Roberts (2005) described four areas of communication breakdown between patients whose first language was not English and their English-speaking general practice physicians. First, there were miscommunications due to variations in stress and intonational contours. Second, there were communication breakdowns due to vocabulary usage or unfamiliarity. Third, there were communication difficulties due to differing narrative styles of patients with non-English cultural backgrounds—their narrative sequences were structured differently. Finally was the problem of differing agendas between the physician and the patient. This last observation is a common area of miscommunication between patients and clinicians regardless of whether linguistic-cultural backgrounds are shared or not.

Traditionally, single case stories or clinical anecdotes are used as illustrations or to identify rare occurrences in medicine, but rarely are they given particular weight in clinical practice. This tendency to dismiss anecdotal—or story—evidence may be one of the reasons why the patient's presenting story, as she comes in to be seen, may not be given the attention it deserves. The lack of attention to patients' stories is compounded by time and economic pressures.

But the patient's version of the health circumstances is critical to understanding the most important issues for dealing with the disorder in general, and to facilitating therapeutic change and/or compliance for that particular patient.

> A story about a problematic issue in health not only tells us what one of the participants experiences, but also entails the claim that this experience is relevant for the issue at stake, and that the issue can be adequately evaluated only if this experience is taken into account and integrated into a practice that aims to deal with the concrete situation (Widdershoven & Smits, 1996, p. 280).

Attending to the stories that an individual patient tells about his or her illness provides a means for identifying which metaphors are used by that individual. Metaphors and narrative structure are linked to culture, but are also individually chosen as the patient tells his or her own story. This may provide a glimpse into how that individual is experiencing the illness. Using the patient's own selected metaphors for coping with the illness or disability provides a framework for personalizing and more effectively individualizing patient care (Casey & Long, 2002).

The discourse of health professionals in regards to stroke and the renegotiation of identity after stroke has been identified as a potential contributor to ultimate stroke outcome. Anderson and Marlett (2004) conceptually link how health professionals talk about living with stroke to potential outcomes. They note that clinicians often focus on ensuring that patients and families have realistic expectations, but patients and their families generally complain about negativity in the discourses and a sense of hopelessness. Discussing possibilities for reconceptualizing one's identity and one's lifestyle after stroke and adaptation to chronic disabilities associated with stroke, such as cognitive-communicative impairments, is recommended as an important aspect of health professional discourse with patients.

For example, I once worked with a client who, any time he said or wrote something which he believed to be an incorrect word choice or incorrectly spelled word, would mutter "Stupid!" to himself. In this case, it was not a great mystery for me to see how this client was thinking of himself.

On the other hand, I once worked with a gentleman who was always very pleasant and controlled, in demeanor an "ideal client." I will never forget the day when this man, contemplating a warm-up activity that he had successfully done in the past, suddenly broke down in uncontrolled sobs. Up until the moment that I sat next to him moving the Kleenex box nearer to him I had never suspected the emotional turmoil he was experiencing. Perhaps he really had not offered me any clues about his emotional state; or perhaps in my glee to be working with such a wonderful client, I had missed them.

A teenage client who had experienced a traumatic brain injury was describing his current speech therapy to me; I was seeing him as part of a second opinion evaluation. He described his computer-based therapy program this way: "You know how if you go to the video arcade every day and play the same game, your score goes up? That's what I do in speech therapy."

Our clients communicate to us their inner experiences. Even a narrative about what a client did over the weekend can have important meaning. The client who simply responds "Nuthin" to such a request for information may be communicating a number of possible meanings. Perhaps this client felt that he or she had nothing to do; the client may be experiencing an acute sense of social isolation. Perhaps the client believes that she has nothing that she *can* do and is experiencing a sense of worthlessness. Alternatively, the client may just be responding normally because she is between the ages of 10 and 17 years!

When we continue to see a client for regular sessions over a period of time, a clinical relationship develops in which roles become established and interaction patterns are formed. Part of the development of a clinical relationship is the growth of emotional regard one for the other between the clinician and the client. Transference is the process in which the client's emotional responses towards others in life are transferred to the clinician. The opposite also occurs; countertransference is the transfer of previously experienced emotional reactions of the clinician to the client. Both of these routine clinical phenomena are described and investigated most actively in clinical psychology, but these processes can occur in any situation in which a clinician and client enter into a therapeutic relationship.

A frequently-cited explanation for transference and countertransference comes from Freudian theory and analysis. An alternative that is more consistent with a social constructionist view comes from a social cognitive approach. In this view, transference (and also countertransference) is seen as the activation of previously stored knowledge structures that are used to help process new elements in the environment. In this case, the new elements include the clinician (or client) as a new character in one's self-narrative and the developing therapeutic relationship (Singer & Singer, 1994). Narrative analysis could provide a more elaborated glimpse into transference and countertransference in the clinical process as they are played out in speech-language pathology.

Beyond our emotional reactions to our clients, clinicians bring their own metaphors and perspectives into narrative construction in the clinical process. Our work settings provide their own meta-narratives and cultural contexts. The vocabulary used in work settings varies; those employed by either schools or hospitals, for example, use different vocabularies to describe the person with the communication disability (e.g., student, patient), the name of the communication disorder, and our evaluation and intervention activities. Beyond differences in vocabulary, different work settings imply a different meta-narrative. In an educational context, for example, the overarching narrative may be one of a student with different abilities who needs individualized supports to achieve educational goals. In a medical context, the story is one of a sick person who is striving to recover and get "back to normal." The work culture infuses itself into our own narrative and how we talk with our clients.

Professional acculturation is important, necessary, and efficient. We may become so adapted to our professional culture that we are no longer consciously aware of how our narrative reflects the meta-narrative of the workplace, and how this relates to our client's narrative. Take, for example, the story of a young woman who, in psychotherapy, retold the sequence of events of her life and everyday experience, but never told stories in which she figured as the protagonist. The activities and cast of characters were described but her role in the events and her reactions to the events were not part of her narrative. It became clear over the course of psychotherapy that this woman was the main character in a story that was being narrated by her mother—acting out someone else's story, rather than creating her own story. Josselson (2004) admonishes therapists to watch for the pitfall of narrating the client's life.

This is a potential risk for speech-language pathologists, as well—such a challenging line to walk when our job is precisely to guide the words, sounds, or communication tools our clients use to tell their story, without unduly influencing the story that they wish to tell!

It is also a potential risk for family members of our clients. Family members, although well-intentioned, can at times be overly zealous in attempting to create a life story for our client that is not really the client's own story for him- or herself. Thus the client is placed in the role of acting out a life story that is being narrated by the family member.

The vulnerability that brings someone in contact with the health system may be precisely the same vulnerability that hampers the client's ability to self-narrate distinctly, or to participate actively in the clinical process. This difficulty is illustrated poignantly by the story of a physician who, requiring treatment for his own serious illness, sought out the most reputable surgeon in the area for his care (Sharf, 2005). As the medical relationship progressed, the patient noted that surgical expertise was not sufficient for the health care process. The patient is in need of a physician who will implement the treatment well, but who is also available for patient consultation and information. Sharf also notes how his own illness, with its resulting decrease in energy and endurance, hampered his ability to actively participate in the clinical care process. He concludes that active patient involvement is encumbered by both the realities of serious illness and the dominant traditional medical model.

How clinicians talk with patients reveals the narrative of the dominant service model, the roles that are being played out by both clinician and client, and the interaction strategies used by both in this context. These sociolinguistic relationships have been successfully investigated by exploring how doctors talk with patients. The typical physician-patient encounter has traditionally been identified in segments: the initial section during which the complaints and reason for the visit are identified; the physical examination; and finally the informational portion of the interaction in which the physician educates the patient as to the nature of the problem and its treatment. Discourse and conversation analysis has been frequently used as a tool to reveal the sociolinguistics of a doctor-patient encounter (Maynard & Heritage, 2005). Discourse markers and features are consistent with the social and authoritative roles ascribed to the doctor and the patient.

Speech-language pathologists have much less frequently turned their own skill in analyzing speech and language onto themselves and their own talk during clinician-client interactions. Leahy (2004) encourages speech-language pathologists to use discourse and conversation analysis, and other ethnographic methods, to analyze the power relationships, linguistic modeling, and social interaction patterns within therapy sessions.

Each component of a typical doctor-patient interaction has been studied using conversation analysis and related ethnographic techniques (Heritage & Maynard, 2005).

In the "opening sequence" of doctor-patient encounters, for example, conversation analysis has been used to identify matches and mismatches between patient and doctor as the patient identifies problem areas, symptoms, or needs. Beginning with the doctor's opening statement, such as "How are you?" or "What can I do for you?" patient and doctor negotiate the nature of their relationship, and how the health problem will be addressed. The physician's opening marks the type of appointment (new problem, follow-up, chronic care). Patients are sensitive to these different types of openings in their responses. When a misalignment occurs between doctor and patient in this opening sequence, concordance in regards to the treatment will be difficult if not impossible to achieve. In other words, patients are unlikely to adhere to a treatment when they are unconvinced that the doctor has clearly understood their complaint or self-identified need (Gafaranga & Britten, 2003).

How well do speech-language pathologists make their own clients feel understood in regards to their self-identified communication problem? In the Gafaranga and Britten (2003) study, and many others like it, the research methodology includes not only conversation analysis of the audiorecorded and transcribed consultation, but also interviews of patient and doctor about their perceptions of the encounter. In this way, stated perceptions after a consultation can be mapped onto the details of the recorded conversation. Identification of the problem to be addressed in a clinician-client relationship is negotiated between both parties, and the relative success of the mutuality of this negotiation may have ramifications for the success of the intervention to follow (Drew & Collins, 2001).

Such an approach could make a nice contribution to our knowledge about the practice of speech-language pathology. Ripich (1989) tells the story of a child describing his experiences in speech therapy. The child explains that it is his "job" in therapy to make the "bad *r*s," and the speech-language pathologist's job in therapy to make the "good *r*s." We need to know as a field what kind of story our clients tell about their experiences during their therapy sessions, and what kind of stories they tell about us as clinicians.

In many medical specialties, studies have been conducted to check back on patients' understanding of what the physician has recommended as appropriate treatment options and associated risks of either treatment or no treatment. This is a critical factor because patients make the ultimate decision about what course to take in regards to any non-emergency medical or health action. A recent example involves a survey of patients' understanding of treatment options in the case of cerebral aneurysm, as presented to them by their vascular surgeon (King, Yonas, Horowitz, Kassam, & Roberts, 2005; Leys, Lejeune, & Pruvo, 2005). Patients completed multiple choice questions and Likert-scale visual analogue items to assess comprehension of best treatment and the risks of various treatments or no treatment. Patients only fairly understood what the best treatment would be in their case, and overestimated the risks of certain treatment options.

This kind of comprehension checking across patients could and should be studied as well in the practice of speech-language pathology. When a parent hears the diagnosis of language-learning disability, how much does that parent understand about the information that was given by the speech-language pathologist? Does she understand the typical intervention course? For those of us who are aphasia clinicians, we observe that clients and their families are often asking basic questions about the aphasia diagnosis in outpatient settings, long after they were first diagnosed and usually after the clients have come into contact with several clinicians. How much was understood at the beginning? What is the trajectory of comprehension about chronic communication disorders over time, and how does comprehension evolve? What communication strategies are most effective for providing initial diagnosis and treatment information to our clients?

Speech-language pathologists know, of course, that comprehension of diagnosis-related information alone is not sufficient to produce a well-informed or well-managed client. The client's affective state and emotional perceptions must also be attended with appropriate responses, and this is accomplished primarily through nonverbal communication within the interaction (see Gallagher, Hartung, Herzina, Gregory, & Merolla, 2005, for an example of a nonverbal communication scale for doctor-patient communication). A recent study of doctor-patient communication linked analysis of the doctor-patient interaction with patients' anxiety levels before and after the appointment. Doctors who provided more adequate information were not necessarily perceived as more empathic by their patients, suggesting that emotional concerns of a patient cannot be met sufficiently with cognitive or informational responses by the physician. Furthermore, patients who perceived that their physician was more empathic reported lower levels of anxiety after the medical encounter (Van Dulmen & van den Brink-Muinen, 2004).

This study of doctor-patient communication demonstrates that there are different potential outcomes in any clinician-client interaction or information exchange. Outcomes of informational exchanges can be described as cognitive, behavioral, or affective (Hinckley, 2000; Hinckley, Craig, & Anderson, 1989). Patients can receive information and understand it—a cognitive outcome—but not necessarily experience lower levels of anxiety—an affective outcome. Presumably the reverse is also possible. Finally, in order to achieve a behavioral outcome—compliance and adherence to a practice regimen or some other behavior change—the client must not only understand the information but must feel that the clinician has adequately understood her complaints and needs and the recommended intervention, therefore, is the right solution for her situation.

For example, interruptions have been studied between physicians and patients. Physicians are more likely to interrupt patients than the reverse; however, men are more likely to interrupt women regardless of the women's role in the encounter—physician or patient (e.g., Rowland-Morin & Carroll, 1990; C. West, 1984). Does this pattern occur in clinical situations in speech-language pathology, when clients are more likely to be male and clinicians are more likely to be female? To my knowledge this kind of discourse analysis of the social dynamics of the clinical process has not been undertaken in our field.

This is not to say that there are no studies of how clinicians talk with their clients. Simmons-Mackie and Damico (1999) investigated the feedback provided by clinicians to adults with aphasia in language treatment. They observed a traditional cycle in which the clinician made a request of the client, the client responded, and feedback was provided regarding the accuracy of the response. This pattern emphasizes the transactional aspects of the clinical interaction, rather than the interactional aspects.

Simmons-Mackie's observation in this study calls to my mind a quotation about interpretation of individuals' narratives.

> If I say to you, speaking of the wedding I attended last week, "And then there was the most amazing coincidence!" I expect you to reply "Really? What happened?" I will be surprised and not especially pleased if instead you say, "Isn't it interesting how you make ordinary events so dramatic?" To pay attention to speakers' rhetoric seems to rob them of authority. It suggests that narrators do not know what they mean to say or cannot find the way to say it and that someone else—the interpreter—can do a better job (Ochberg, 1996, p. 97).

For some traditional approaches and some clinical circumstances in speech-language pathology, this is exactly our assumption—the clinician is assumed to be able to do a better job and help the client do a better job of saying what the client wants to say. As a result we tend to put our interactional energies on the form and manner in which a client communicates a message. This is, of course, not always true, and many clinicians and particular therapeutic approaches emphasize the message and the communication interaction over the way in which it was communicated. But even then, we tend to praise our clients for finding a way to get the message across, rather than simply responding to their message in a typical social way. More than likely, our clients would find a "normal" conversational response equally encouraging and perhaps even more reinforcing than emphasizing communication forms.

In another study, Simmons-Mackie and Schultz (2003) studied the use of humor in aphasia therapy sessions. They observed that humor was most often used by the clinician to build rapport, facilitate cooperation, or avoid embarrassment. They also observed that humor was almost exclusively used by the clinician, and not initiated by the client. They suggest that equalizing the "humor balance" within a therapy session might serve to change the power dynamics within the clinician-client interaction.

Another area that has been often studied is the use of a simplified speech style by nurses and other caregivers. A simplified speech style is characterized by exaggerated intonation contours, unique and simplified vocabulary items (e.g., *pee-pee* for *urination*), and short utterance lengths. These speech style characteristics are often found in speech directed to children by their caregivers, as well as in the speech directed to elderly patients by their caregivers. When simplified speech is directed towards an older adult, it usually implies condescension and incompetence, whether the speaker intends it or not. In some instances, however, it is viewed positively by some listeners as conveying nurturing.

I doubt that speech-language pathologists are at risk for an indiscriminate use of such a simplified speech style. It would seem, on the contrary, that our training inoculates us against its use. Certainly there are dimensions of modifying speech styles that speech-language pathologists are trained to use, and we are trained to vary modifications in speech style from one client need to another. The implementation of speech style modifications in actual practice by experienced clinicians has not, to my knowledge, been systematically observed. Such a study might give us insight as to whether we really do lengthen response opportunities as long as we think we do; how effectively we really are in maintaining eye gaze with our clients during communication breakdowns; and how some of our own clinical discourse behaviors are perceived by our clients.

Another potential area for additional research in clinician-client discourse in speech-language pathology is to analyze the discourse that occurs during information-giving or counseling. Hersch (2001) used in-depth interviewing in a qualitative research study to describe the discharge strategies used by speech-language pathologists ending therapy for clients with aphasia. Interviews revealed that clients were not necessarily clear on the reasons why therapy ended and clinicians may be ambivalent or conflicted about having to discharge the clients. Clinicians may be facing caseload pressures or reimbursement justification pressures that are difficult for clients to comprehend. Clients may be reluctant to ask for clarification about why a therapist stops seeing them. Furthermore, Hersch (2001) observed that the medical record did not reflect all of the reasons taken into consideration by the clinician for the discharge. Five categories of discharge strategies were observed by Hersch (2003): wait-and-see, negotiation, preparation, separation, and replacement. Weaning may be a process by which therapists attempt to have clients move on to other activities besides formal therapy while maintaining their therapeutic relationship.

This kind of research should be extended to other aspects of the clinical process and clinician-client discourse. If we made observations of typical clinical information exchanges, how understandable is the information that we provide? How clear? How short are our sentences, how long our pauses? Do we not only provide opportunities for questions but facilitate them? What discourse features exist in our counseling sessions that mirror other counseling domains, or incorporate typically effective counseling discourse techniques? The analysis of our own clinician-client discourse has the potential to reveal much about the effectiveness of our interactions with clients, and can also expose the inner workings of our clinical relationships with our clients.

The interaction and communication skills of a clinician may affect specific clinical outcomes in important ways. A simple intervention that has been described in the context of doctor-patient communication involves patient question-asking (Wells, Falk, & Dieppe, 2004). Patients are specifically asked to write out questions and discussion topics for the doctor in advance of a medical encounter. The doctors perceived these questions and topics as a very helpful way to appreciate the current understanding of the patients regarding specific medical issues. Patients perceive the ability to focus their questions and issues in advance, and having them addressed in the medical encounter, as highly desirable and improving satisfaction. Such a simple but powerful approach may also improve adherence to prescribed regimens or practice.

Narrative between Clinicians

If we define and create images of our own identities with narrative, then the narratives we create with other professionals must equally contribute to our professional identities. These narratives are embedded not only in a broad cultural context but also in the culture of our profession, and the more localized culture of our individual workplace. Elements of our professional narratives will relate to these cultural contexts, and be consistent with them. The use of stories is not just to conform and confirm our membership in the broader cultural contexts, including our professional context, but also to distinguish ourselves as individuals within that context. Speech-language pathologists who work in the Hillsborough County

School District in Tampa, Florida, share many aspects of their professional context. But within the particular constraints and processes of that workplace, each speech-language pathologist must identify his or her niche. So within narratives about our work we will find themes reflecting cultural commonalities and events or reactions that highlight individual differences.

When It's "Just Us": Clinicians Only

Narratives between clinicians include stories about the workplace and stories about our clinical interactions and efforts. We tell stories to each other about what happened when we talked to so-and-so, and how that meeting was different than when a colleague met with the same colleague. We complain about new documentation regulations or pass on helpful hints about how to negotiate regulatory issues. Stories about the workplace serve to express our emotions, form professional bonds, and sometimes pass on useful information.

We also tell stories to each other about our work with clients. We share with colleagues the reactions we had to parents or other family members, or how we managed (or mismanaged) a particularly challenging emotional response on the part of a client or client's family member. We express our pride about our successes, and our doubts and disappointments about our daily work that we think could have been improved. When we are unsure, we tell the story to a professional friend and ask for another alternative to what we did. These stories serve not only the goals of emotional expression, sharing, and forming professional bonds, but also serve as an informal means of peer review. When our particular employment setting does not provide formalized means of peer review of our own clinical work, we seek out informal ones by sharing clinical stories with a trusted colleague.

By sharing stories with our colleagues, we co-create meaning from our daily professional events. For speech-language pathologists, this may occur in a lunchroom or at the end of the day during a paperwork time, when clinicians are in their offices. For nurses, the nursing station has been characterized as the "storytelling center" in a medical clinical context. It forms a location where social interaction creates meaning out of the events of the clinic (Morgan-Witte, 2005).

These stories between us as clinicians have been little if ever attended to in our public and professional dialogue. In contrast, stories that doctors and nurses tell to each other have been thought about for what they reveal about the medical workplace and its culture, as well as how individual clinicians cope with the unusual clinical situations in which they find themselves. The purposes of the professional discourse are many, and there is probably a wealth of knowledge about our own profession that could be revealed by a systematic analysis and discussion of the stories we tell each other.

It's not just the telling of the stories, but also the listening and the kind of responses that are offered by colleagues that create and reveal meaning. Sometimes humor is used as a way to lighten situations, or distance ourselves from difficult circumstances. At other times we may not know what to say, and our responses may tend to reiterate the standards of the professional culture in which we find ourselves.

A case example is reported in the literature of an elementary school teacher who told a story to different audiences about a disagreement involving her, a parent, and her principal (Whelan, Huber, Rose, Davies, & Clandinin, 2001). When she told the story to a group of her fellow teachers, she received agreement with her own position but no challenges to her own thinking or alternatives to consider. When she told the story to other groups, including fellow professionals outside of her immediate teaching circle, she received support for considering different perspectives about the situation. Telling the story to other professionals served as a means for affirming her position, in one context, but also supported the consideration of other perspectives. Although it is not specifically discussed by Whelan and colleagues. (2001), these new interactions very likely affected the way in which the teacher subsequently retold the same story.

A recently published book by Katharine Weber (2006) centers on the power of repeating a self-defining anecdote. The book is about the oldest survivor of the Triangle shirtwaist factory fire in 1911, Rose Freeman, who died in 2001 at the age of 107. The novel is based on interviews and transcripts of how Ms. Freeman retold the story of surviving the fire, maintaining a certain level of notoriety all of her life based on this single event. The story of the fire and the night she didn't die is retold to different people, in different contexts, evolving over time. Stories are reconstructed as they are retold (Mishler, 2004). Stories do indeed have the power to define us—and the stories we tell each other as clinicians can also define us as therapists.

Our Clients, Ourselves

The stories we choose to tell to colleagues are selected based on what is appropriate in the cultural context, and also based on the nature of the relationship we have with a particular colleague. Without a doubt, there are stories about our clinical work that we tell only to ourselves—in quiet moments, maybe during the drive home, when we reflect on a moment with a client that had no other witnesses, and we ask ourselves honestly if we couldn't have handled it better than we did. Such a critical introspection is part of the process of continuous improvement and professional development. When we reflect on other events that affect us, perhaps outside of our professional lives, linking these experiences back to the experiences of our clients will make us more sensitive and attuned to our clients. Even physicians have been encouraged to write expressively and creatively about their own experiences, in prose or poetry, as a mechanism in which they become more attuned to their own inner experiences. It has been argued that this will allow them to be more sensitive to the inner experiences of their patients (Stein, 2004).

Internal dialogue or reflections about our professional selves and informal conversations with colleagues about professional events are fundamental to our professional existence and development. These stories become part of a more formal professionwide dialogue when they are shared in classrooms and workshops. Typically, however, these stories of clinical experience are used as illustrations and are often not really even part of a main outline of an instructional talk or presentation. It is possible to make these professional experiences more of our professionwide formal discourse, by adopting a narrative-based approach to practice and applying it equally to the clinician side of the therapy equation. If clinical interactions are constructed by the interaction of the clinician and the client, then stories focused on us as clinicians—our emotional responses, our reactions, our perspectives—must be equally revealing to understanding and learning about the clinical process as are stories focused on the client. Both kinds of stories—those focused on the experience and responses of the clinician, and those focused on the experience and responses of the client—are an important means to develop clinicians—pre-professionally and professionally. All of these kinds of stories warrant a place in our public, professional discussion.

Narrative and the Development of a Speech-Language Pathologist

Speech-language pathologists benefit from the stories of their colleagues. During our early training, we listen with rapt attention to the stories of our instructors and supervisors about their clinical experiences. We tell stories to our fellow students about our own clinical experiences. As we gain professional experience, we are still equally interested in listening to and telling stories about our work. These stories can be an informal means of professional development and training, and they can also be a more formalized technique in training and professional development. When they become more public we tend to refer to these stories as anecdotes, and when we incorporate anecdotes systematically into our teaching efforts, it is referred to as case-based (or problem-based) learning. In any form, talking about our learning, and in particular making stories about our learning, facilitates lifelong development (Pamphilon, 2005).

Narrative and the Development of Reflection

It has been observed that there are strong analogies between the student clinician-supervisor relationship and the clinician-client relationship (Milan, Parish, & Reichgott, 2006). So tools and techniques that are used to teach clinical skills may very well be internalized and applied to the student clinician's future relationships with clients as well as future supervisees. In one example, clinical communication skills typically relied on in the clinical encounter were applied to the supervisory training interaction (Milan, Parish, & Reichgott, 2006). Skills used to develop rapport and effective clinician-client relationships in the clinical interaction are used to provide feedback and support to student clinicians. The model also incorporated the use of the stage of readiness to change (SOC) model to help the supervisor determine when the student clinician was ready to address particular clinical skills to be improved. Stages of readiness to change are thought to be important aspects of behavior change, and include assessments about whether an individual is considering behavior change, intending to change in the near future, or actively planning to change (Prochaska & DiClemente, 1984; Prochaska, 1994; Prochaska & Velicer, 1997; but for a criticism of the model, see R. West, 2005).

Another approach to training good clinician-client communication skills comes from the realm of medical student training. In this approach, it was also observed that good supervisor-student communication skills are similar to those used in patient care. Since supervisors are expert clinicians themselves, this observation facilitates the application of already developed communication skills in the supervisors. At the same time, the use of an organized communication system to provide feedback and instruction to student clinicians helps to model and foster the communication skills that the students will use with clients. The approach developed by Kern et al. (2005) is summarized by the acronym CAARE MORE. These letters represent the following concepts: connect personally with the trainee; ask psychosocial questions; assess the trainee's knowledge, attitudes, skills, and behaviors; role model desired attitudes, skills, and behaviors; create a safe, supportive, enjoyable learning environment; formulate specific management strategies regarding psychosocial issues; observe the trainee's affect and behavior; reflect and provide feedback on doctor-patient and preceptor-trainee interactions; and provide educational resources and best evidence. The CAARE MORE model and similar training approaches emphasize the matching of the training communication environment to client-clinician communication skills that are used in the clinical interaction.

The use of narrative approaches and narrative reflection has also been incorporated into clinical supervision, and aids student clinicians to incorporate personal experience of all types into their developing professional persona (Harper, 2004). This facilitates the integration of new knowledge about clinical procedures into already existing knowledge that has been accumulated from general world experience.

In fact, the Declarative, Procedural, and Reflective (DPR) model is a cognitive model of the development of therapist skills (Bennett-Levy, 2006). This model acknowledges and describes the role of declarative knowledge, procedural knowledge, and reflection in the development of therapist expertise. The declarative knowledge portion of this model includes the conceptual knowledge about clinical work. The procedural knowledge includes understanding about how and when to implement particular treatments. The reflection portion of this model incorporates clinicians' ability to reflect on their own declarative and procedural knowledge as well as their own self and personal reactions as they pertain to and are incorporated into their professional role. This is one example of a model of the development of therapist skill that places reflection in a central and pivotal role.

Recent examples using literary texts in medical training and other health-related pre-professional training demonstrate how discussions of nonscientific texts can improve sensitivity and clinical communication skills. For example, the use of nontraditional sources that address issues of living with illness, disability, death, and dying enables student clinicians to imagine themselves in such a story, thus increasing identification and empathy (Wear & Aultman, 2005).

In a specific medical training example, pediatric residents participated in a monthly discussion group with staff members of an inner-city Dominican-American community organization (DasGupta, Meyer, Calero-Breckheimer, Costley, & Guillen, 2006). Literary texts were discussed, rather than case studies. The authors argue that the discussion of literary texts provided a context in which the members of the two groups could discuss cultural similarities and differences and appreciate different interpretations and perspectives to the discussed text. Qualitative data analysis suggested that members of both groups improved in their appreciation of cultural diversity and understanding of medical culture. Both groups also were helped to explore physicians' attitudes and beliefs about medical practice and how cultural issues impact health care.

Narrative-based approaches have been incorporated even more directly into clinical training examples by some. For example, Gaver, Borkan, & Weingarten (2005) used a narrative approach to developing clinical sensitivity and clinical communication skills among second-year medical students in Tel Aviv. Each student was matched with a volunteer family in the community who was living with a chronic medical condition. The student met with the family five times per year, and produced narrative essays in which they were expected to reflect on their experiences with patients as teachers. The students learned to listen to the patients' narratives in a family context, and also met in small groups with an instructor to enhance learning and reflection. Some of the outcomes of this approach were an increase in understanding the role of the family in managing patient care, learning to adopt a nonpatronizing and nonjudgmental attitude, and developing specific communication skills.

An even more personalized approach to training integration of personal experience with clinical experience is demonstrated by the incorporation of personal illness stories into medical education (DasGupta & Charon, 2004). Students were asked to write their own narrative about a personal illness experience, thus providing an opportunity for the students to reflect specifically and explicitly on their own emotional reactions and experiences to being ill. The underlying premise is that bringing these experiences to conscious awareness and linking them to the clinical training process will facilitate empathy and sensitivity in the clinical interaction.

Some training programs have characterized their entire first-year clinical skills program as *narrative structuring* (Pullman, Bethune, & Duke, 2005). In this work, the clinical interaction is characterized explicitly as the writing of and participation in one another's stories. Students are asked to write narratives and reflective essays on assigned literary texts and ethical practice in relation to specific case studies. Students also maintain journals of their clinical reflections. Students are explicitly expected to think about the story that is being told by the patient and is being created by the interaction of the client and clinician in the clinical process.

Reflection when one's training is complete is also a productive exercise. In a collection of autobiographical essays (Takakuwa, Rubashkin, & Herzig, 2004), recent medical graduates wrote about their personal struggles and summed up "what I learned in medical school." Some of these essays demonstrate the difficulty of integrating personal experience and identity into a fairly rigid training system that emphasized analytical processes.

Of course, studies incorporating narrative-based approaches to clinical training are not limited to medical school. Literary accounts of experiences in aging or illness can serve to educate future allied health professionals as well (Nuessel & Van Stewart, 1999). It has also been shown that producing narratives about externship placements can facilitate the integration of learning among speech-language pathology students (Cortazzi, Jin, Wall, & Cavendish, 2001). These narratives, when shared with peers or instructors, can consolidate learning, enhance professional confidence, and help to foster a shared narrative about what is expected and experienced by those at that stage of their training.

The use of reflective writing in clinical training of various kinds is not a novel idea, of course. But the usefulness of the application of various forms of narrative into clinical training is being acknowledged for its specific outcomes. We know that, in asking questions about treatment for communication disorders, the question is not "Which treatment is best?" but rather, "Which treatment is appropriate for which client to achieve which outcome?" Similarly, in developing clinical expertise recent work points to the understanding that analytical training focused on procedural knowledge produces the mechanical skills of being a clinician, but narrative-based approaches in training yield integrative skills including empathy, sensitivity, and clinical communication abilities. Empathy is linked to narrative (Schafer, 2004). A number of different training activities and models are being developed in health professions, and these approaches are likely to increase in prevalence and become more refined as they are addressed systematically for effectiveness and specific outcomes.

Clinical Anecdotes

From the point of view of evidence-based practice, clinical anecdotes are a very weak form of evidence on which to make clinical decisions, such as selecting an appropriate treatment (Hinckley, 2007). Hunter (1986) refers to the "pejorative cloud that hangs over anecdote" because of the real risk of drawing broad conclusions from a single case or a small group of cases. In spite of this danger, anecdote persists as a phenomenon in all clinical situations.

Anecdotes fit into evidence-based practice when previously unknown clinical presentations arise. In this case, the best and only way to begin a professional dialogue about the clinical picture is to share the story of a single case. Beyond evidence-based practice, however, clinical anecdotes are a routine part of any professional's life. We heard them starting in our training classrooms and we continue to be interested in them and share stories about individual clinical experiences throughout our careers. Clinical anecdotes hold a certain power because they are persuasive and instructive in a way that general conclusions from an evidence-based approach cannot be; they illustrate details, intentions, and lived experiences in a way that brings general guidelines to life. Anecdotes serve some basic educational purposes within a clinical setting. First, they make points easier to remember; a story about a case is a good mnemonic. Anecdotes are also good illustrations of major points. They can serve as cautionary tales and report mistakes that should not be repeated. They can also illustrate by sharing the story of a counterexample.

Anecdotes also serve to form professional bonds within groups of colleagues. According to Hunter (1986), "the smaller the group and the more similar their clinical activities, the more anecdotes will be told." Such stories will likely share a great deal of common knowledge among a group of practitioners, and also reflect their specific work setting and culture. Anecdotes within a particular practice setting also aid individuals in creating meaning about their daily work and the clinical events of the day—either routine or nonroutine.

Anecdotes also provide a route for handling failure. When a clinical situation does not go as expected, telling the story of the events to colleagues can serve to work out a perceived misstep, and help the clinician make sense of the sequence of events leading to its end.

Anecdotes come in various forms. A full, formalized case presentation is one form of clinical anecdote. At the other extreme are half-sentences, such as "I've seen that" (Hunter, 1986, p. 625), to acknowledge an unusual presentation. Anecdotes can be affirmative, illustrating that a certain event or combination of events can happen clinically. Anecdotes can also serve comparative functions, to contrast a current case with a recollected case, for example.

Finally, anecdotes help us to learn how to be good clinicians. We understand more about our colleagues' intentions and subsequent actions by listening to their stories. We imagine ourselves in their circumstances, and consider what our own actions might or might not have been.

The clinician-in-training is especially in need of hearing clinical anecdotes. Clinicians set out to be good; but in so doing, they must look around and ask themselves "What is a good clinician?" "Who, specifically, do I want to be like?" Stories from both less experienced and more experienced clinicians allow the developing clinician to project oneself into the story, considering whether the same actions or responses would have been made, and if different, how or why they would have been different.

Describing the importance of fairy tales to the development of the self in children, Bettelheim wrote:

> The question for the child is not "Do I want to be good?" but "Who do I want to be like?" The child decides this on the basis of projecting himself wholeheartedly into one character. If this fairy tale figure is a very good person, then the child decides that he wants to be good, too (Bettelheim, 1976, p. 10).

This argument holds true for the development of a professional persona. It is well accepted that pre-professional clinicians often take on stylistic variations of their supervisors, trying them on like outfits, keeping parts of one and something else from another. This process continues until there are no more supervisors—there are peers and colleagues, and we do not often observe each other doing the thing we most want to do well. We are left to perform self-analysis and learn from our interactions with our clients.

Case-Based Learning

In all levels of formal education, narrative forms have been emphasized as a way to facilitate memory and learning, and to impact students' everyday lives. Narrative psychology has been used as a background and rationale for the use of story development in educational settings. Gleaning new information expressed in the context of a personal story facilitates both storage and retrieval of new information. Computer technology, including the Internet and hypertext, which supports such expressive tools as Web pages and blogs, facilitates the rapid development of personal stories integrating information gleaned from Internet and computer sources and expressed in a computer environment (Berg, 2000).

Learning of textbook material is also enhanced through narrative. When college students are exposed to either narrative-style material or traditionally presented material in an introductory psychology course, narrative facilitated retrieval of the information both in the short and long term. Additionally, students expressed a preference for the narrative style material (Fernald, 1987; 1994). Students learn better, even in a typical university course, if material is presented and tested in a narrative mode (Fernald, 1994). When training future allied health professionals, literary accounts of experiences in aging or illness can serve as powerful examples and an important schema for information retrieval (Nuessel & Van Stewart, 1999).

A formalized technique for incorporating clinical scenarios into professional training is case-based or problem-based learning (PBL). PBL has become a viable pedagogical technique in medical and allied health training. PBL is an educational approach that is learner centered. The learner, in conjunction with a learning group of fellow students and a facilitator, sets out to identify and then learn relevant clinical knowledge that pertains to a presented case. A curriculum committee or other similar group develops a set of cases that will facilitate coverage of key clinical knowledge areas.

PBL can be differentiated from traditional clinical teaching (Dornan, Scherpbier, King, & Boshuizen, 2005): Traditionally, the teacher sets the pace and determines the content of the learning environment. In PBL, the learner self-determines need areas. Traditional methods are didactic and authoritarian; in PBL the teacher is facilitative. In PBL, a curriculum committee or other group determines the curriculum by setting up exemplar cases so that students are exposed to various clinical scenarios and knowledge areas. Traditional clinical teaching was unsystematic and determined largely on what patients came through the clinic during a student's rotation, and what the instructor thought to highlight or teach regarding each case. Traditional clinical teaching emphasizes professional tasks and roles, whereas PBL foregrounds student knowledge and skills. In PBL, the source of information is private study and the student's peers in discussion and learning groups; traditionally, the source of information is the teacher with some private study on the part of the student.

It has been argued that PBL is an appropriate educational approach to consider in audiology, since training in audiology shares many of the expectations for medical and related professional training (Tharpe, Rassi, & Biswas, 1995). By now, programs in other allied health disciplines such as physical therapy and some speech-language pathology programs have adopted PBL across the curriculum. Where this has occurred, the benefits of narrative are built into the entire curriculum systematically. Students increase their problem-solving abilities, including research skills and peer review and discussion. Students in a PBL approach also benefit from hearing the same set of stories, each story providing a coherent, detailed illustration of general guidelines. PBL builds on the mnemonic strengths of stories while showing students how cases begin and end and how clinicians respond to sets of realistic circumstances. Thus, general guidelines and details of lived experiences are linked from the beginning of training. In contrast, traditional approaches typically expect students to learn general conclusions, waiting months or a year before they are truly exposed to a complete clinical case presentation that is linked to that general concept.

Narrative and Clinical Errors

In recent years, the health care establishment has turned its attention to the role of clinical incidents and errors: causes, prevention, and their disclosure on the part of health care workers. In many states, licensure requires specific training in medical and clinical errors. This is a result of the understanding that prevention of medical errors requires a culture that tolerates disclosure and discussion of errors in a nonblaming way. More education about the roots and management of errors is thought to facilitate acknowledgement of errors and compliance with error and incident reporting policies.

Error seems to be as human as narrative. One of the uses of narrative in any individual's life story is the reflection of perceived wrongs or mistakes and the integration of those actions or inactions into the rest of one's life story. It is not surprising, then, that narrative approaches have been applied to analyzing clinical incidents and medical errors.

Narratives provide a way to make meaning from events, so producing a narrative about a potential or actual clinical error can help the individual and the institution make sense from events leading to the error. Clinical incident reporting requires a description of the setting of the error—people involved, time, and location. It also demands a reporting of what happened, often done in a narrative format. These narratives require a sharing of the self, emotional experiences in the clinical setting, and responses to specific clinical incidents in a way that has not previously been the case (Iedema,

Flabouris, Grant, & Jorm, 2006). Clinicians are willing to report patient safety data using narratives as well as other coding schemas, and in fact seem appreciative of the opportunity to produce narratives about reportable incidents (Nast et al., 2005).

Recently, a narrative approach has been taken to analyze the Medicare claims of individuals during the last 3 years prior to their death (Barnato et al., 2005). Claims were reviewed and a clinical narrative was produced by trained abstracters. The narratives revealed issues about quality of life, continuity of care, and possible medical errors. The narratives provided a more in-depth analysis of a series of Medicare claims than a simple analysis of vital statistics.

Narrative enables us to create meaning out of events, and part of that meaning in clinical settings is to reconsider ethical patterns of behavior and to revisit ethical and moral dialogues and dilemmas. Narrative is a commonly used form to teach ethics, for example to students in health-related disciplines, but it is also an important technique for addressing and coping with clinical fallibility (Solbakk, 2004).

In requiring narratives about critical incidents or errors, organizations are infusing narrative practices into at least one routine aspect of health care in a new way. Particularly in medical environments, the work culture often does not facilitate self-disclosure of any kind, really, and particularly not for potential mistakes. Our more systematic analysis of medical errors is an attempt to break down these work culture barriers. Thirty-nine physicians who had been in practice an average of 12 years were asked to write a narrative about medical error in their past. Interestingly, a majority of those physicians reported that they had disclosed the medical error to another physician, a significant other, or a patient (Allman, 1996). The narratives that these physicians wrote about the commission of a medical error also suggested that there was relatively little discussion with others about the emotional effects of the error.

For clinicians to discuss clinical errors in narrative form leads, naturally enough, to clinicians discussing clinical successes in narrative form, as well. If specific training on the root causes and prevention of medical errors is important to continued quality of care, shouldn't specific training on the root causes and facilitation of clinical successes be equally important to continued quality of care?

STUDY/DISCUSSION QUESTIONS AND ACTIVITIES

1. Audio-record a session you have with one of your clients. Analyze it in terms of discourse and conversational features, such as: turn-taking, interruptions, initiations, total time at talk, number of utterances, rate of speech, amount of silence, length of pauses, or other features.
2. Reflect on a story that one of your clients told you—this could be a story about the weekend, about an important life event, or the story of the communication disorder. Are there aspects of this story that you appreciate differently or think differently about upon reflection or in retrospect?
3. Reflect on a story you told a colleague about a client. Think honestly about your own motivations for telling this story. Were you seeking sympathy, approval, or affiliation? How did your colleague respond? What do you think your colleague was communicating to you?

15

The Growth of a Client

OVERVIEW

In this chapter, three examples of intervention approaches that are built on a narrative approach are described. First, social and personal outcomes of the use of personal narrative are described. Second, therapeutic writing paradigms are explored for possible clinical applications. Finally, the literature on bibliotherapy is reviewed with possible implications for speech-language pathology.

LEARNING OBJECTIVES

At the end of this chapter, the reader will be able to:

1. Identify one way to integrate personal narrative into an intervention approach.

2. List two possible nonlinguistic outcomes of the use of personal narratives in intervention.

3. Describe the application of either bibliotherapy or a therapeutic writing paradigm to intervention in speech-language pathology.

Direct Benefits of Narrative to the Client

Approaches to narrative-based practice provide clinicians ways to integrate evidence-based guidelines and standards with individual circumstances during clinical decision making. Narratives about the clinical process also bring attention to the emotional and social interactive aspects of the clinical relationship, including clinical discourse, that are otherwise difficult to explore and study. Both of these broad areas of narrative application offer indirect benefits to clients, by enlarging the scope of formal and public clinical discussion of these topics and making them explicit. Narrative-based practice can also point to directions of clinical activities that have the potential to offer direct benefit to the client. There are numerous ideas and future directions for narrative applications in working with clients, and many of these remain to be developed more fully and shared with the profession. In this chapter, I use the existing literature on this topic to outline some broad areas of potential clinical applications of narrative-based practice.

Personal Narrative in Intervention

Personal narratives are frequently used in intervention, of course. The telling of personal stories is a highly relevant and personally important thing to do. In what follows I would like to describe three interesting applications of personal narrative that highlight the integration of narrative skills with an acknowledgement of personal growth and self-identity in the clinical process.

First, personal narratives can have social outcomes beyond the improvement of linguistic abilities or the production of narrative structures. Narratives are an important means by which clients develop new stories about themselves and their new roles as they live with a communication disorder. The recent growth in the publication of personal narratives of all sorts—and in their recognition in an ever-widening circle that includes people without experience with a disorder (and also professionals)—demonstrates how important narratives are to the development of meaning.

For example, a recent issue of the magazine of the American Speech-Language-Hearing Association (*ASHA Leader*) featured the personal narrative of a gentleman with amyotrophic lateral sclerosis (ALS) (Portnuff, 2006). He writes about his own experiences with communication strategies including augmentative-assistive communication (AAC) techniques and devices. His purpose in writing the article published in this magazine was to provide speech-language pathologists with insights from a consumer that might help SLPs develop appropriate communication strategies for other clients with speech disorder due to ALS. His sister, a speech-language pathologist, also wrote a sidebar to the article about her experiences using specific communication strategies. In this case, at least one purpose of the personal narrative was to help others in a similar situation by increasing understanding and knowledge of speech-language pathologists. Making a contribution to others in a similar condition requires a degree of acknowledgement of one's own situation and a desire to make a contribution.

The Krempels Brain Injury Foundation Oral History Project has as its goal to facilitate public education and awareness by recording the narratives of individuals living with traumatic brain injury (Fraas & Kalvert, 2006a). These oral histories help to educate students going into allied health professions. The stories are also a powerful resource for helping other people with traumatic brain injury and their families to understand potential sequelae of brain injury and to appreciate that others have dealt with these problems, too. Stories like these can show others what kind of things to expect in the future and provide a sense of hope.

Getting to know a person with a communication disorder by listening to or reading a personal narrative written by that person can promote more positive attitudes towards individuals with communication disorders. For example, personal narratives can promote positive attitudes toward users of AAC who have severe communication disabilities among business majors, who could be expected to be future employers (McCarthy, Donofrio, Dempsey, Birr, & Pratt, 2006).

Production of a narrative about new life behaviors may facilitate adherence to new health regimens such as exercise or medication-taking (McGannon, 2002). Many clients need to develop new communication procedures, strategies, or new speech or swallowing skills. To do so, adherence to a regular practice regimen is needed. Clients with swallowing disorders may need to integrate new eating routines or swallowing strategies; clients with speech disorders may need to make adjustments to increase intelligibility; clients with language disorders may need to use alternative modalities or linguistic strategies to transmit their messages. It is possible that when the client generates a new story about him- or herself that incorporates this new routine, it can facilitate the integration of these new behaviors to a new self-image, thus promoting accommodation and also adherence to the new routine. The observation that narrative facilitates adherence to other health behaviors such as exercise suggests promise for the investigation of narrative as a way to promote adherence to speech, swallowing, or language strategies among our clients with communication disorders.

Autobiographical reports can be used to develop consumer education programs and seminars (Pound, Parr, & Duchan, 2001). Asking support persons of individuals living with aphasia to tell a story about their lives can help clinicians target important areas of continued education and plan relevant support services.

Narrative therapy (described in Chapter 2) as used in stuttering treatment demonstrates an intervention that complements impairment-based therapy by providing a holistic view of the person who stutters (Leahy, 2004). Narrative therapy can help the individual examine the role that the stutter plays in his or her life and think about the roles he or she plays as a person who stutters (DiLollo, Neimeyer, & Manning, 2002; DiLollo, Manning, & Neimeyer, 2003). Tackling these holistic lifestyle issues may make important contributions to the maintenance of therapeutic gain and generalization across contexts within the individual's life.

Therapeutic and Expressive Writing

The many general positive health benefits of narrative were described in Chapter 2. From the literature reviewed in Chapter 2, we learned that the use of narrative in a variety of activities and procedures can produce both physical and psychological health improvements. Narrative appears to facilitate the development and implementation of coping strategies, and improved coping—achieved in any way—is typically associated with positive health benefits.

One of the hypotheses that stems from research linking narrative forms including therapeutic writing to positive health benefits is the cognitive change hypothesis (Pennebaker & Seagal, 1999). Pennebaker and Seagal (1999) suggest that two critical elements must be incorporated into therapeutic writing to facilitate positive outcomes. The first critical element is that the telling of a traumatic or emotional event must be in the form of a story. The story form typically evolves from a set of disjointed perceptions and lends coherence and meaning to the events. The second critical element is that words with emotional content must be used to emotionally process past events and reinterpret them in a positive way. Specifically, vocabulary items associated with *insight* and *causality* have been linked to improved health outcomes; increase in the use of these categories of vocabulary words from the first to the last writing session (over a three to five writing session period) has been associated with fewer doctor visits, improved immune functioning, and positive lifestyle changes (Pennebaker, Mayne, & Francis, 1997).

The challenge to us who work with those with communication disorders is that some of those communication disorders specifically affect the client's ability to formulate a narrative. Does the client's telling of his own story improve as narrative structures and abilities are targeted in intervention? Are these improvements linked to improved coping, adjustment, or other health benefits?

It would be interesting to explore how targeting the story form and vocabulary categories of emotional descriptors might be linked to coping and health among persons with communication disorders. What we know about the development of mental state vocabulary items among children with various types of language disabilities (for example, Naigles, 2001; Dennis, 2001; Johnston, Miller, & Tallal, 2001) might be interesting to link to this type of expressive narrative. Chapter 6 provides a basic overview of how we understand the development of narrative among children with communication disorders and the impairment of narrative abilities among those children and adults with communication disorders due to traumatic onset of illness or injury. We have not yet linked this understanding of narrative and specific vocabulary categories to outcomes other than specific language outcomes.

Indeed, what is needed is to link impairments of narrative or specific vocabulary categories and their improvement to more than impairment-based outcomes. The World Health Organization International Classification of Impairment, Disability, and Handicap (ICIDH-2; ICF, 2001) describes levels of functioning including impairment, activity, and participation. Clinical outcomes associated with the impairment level are those that measure physiological or mental functions, while outcomes associated with activity and participation levels are those that measure, for example, performance of daily activities, social participation, and quality of life. It would be potentially important to explore how improvement in narrative production abilities or the production of specific categories of mental or emotional terms might be linked to physical and psychological health outcomes.

This is perhaps easiest to envision as it might be applied to adults with communication disorders. What would happen if adults with communication disorders participated in a therapeutic writing experience, like the Pennebaker paradigm? Clients might begin with describing the onset of their communication disorder in a relatively disjointed way, but with its retelling might develop in the ability to derive meaning from the event. Those of us who are lucky enough to work with adults living with chronic communication disorder often observe these clients telling and retelling the story of the onset of their communication disorder. This is very likely because they are deriving meaning from doing so and doing it with different conversational partners, creating a slightly different story each time relative to the social context. Could the clinician be instrumental in more assertively facilitating this process, by engaging the client in a series of writing exercises or in telling the story of their communication disorder in an intentionally repetitive and systematic way?

For those clients who are significantly challenged in their linguistic ability to formulate a narrative—even a self-narrative—

options exist that might compensate for the linguistic impairment. Node-link or knowledge maps may produce similar physical and psychological benefits to expressive or narrative writing, and this may be an important avenue to pursue for clients with language disorders who may have difficulty with a traditional therapeutic expressive writing paradigm (Todd, 1999). Another alternative is to produce a narrative through alternative modalities, such as in a portfolio form (Pound, Parr, Lindsay, & Woolf, 2000). It would be interesting to discover whether telling the story of a traumatic event like the onset of a communication disorder in a portfolio format is equally powerful in terms of potential coping and health benefits as telling one's story through therapeutic writing or typical narrative format.

Developing a narrative about one's own disability both reflects current coping state and facilitates the development of coping. Since adjustment to chronic disability is a long-term process, an alternative to the traditional therapeutic writing paradigm over only a few sessions is to develop long-term journaling skills. Journaling can be used for self-expression, self-exploration, and relaxation and can contribute to stress reduction. The key components to journaling are patience, practice, and consistency (Landis, 2004), and thus may coexist positively with the long-term experience of adapting to life with a chronic communication disability. Journaling workbooks are available (e.g., Thomas, 1984; Rich & Copans, 1998) and adaptations of these workbooks could help the clinician to direct a client in developing a journal.

For clients with impairments that limit their ability to engage in a typical written journal, alternative forms may produce equal benefits. Video journals are common now and might prove an effective alternative. Similarly, journals that include drawings, copies of meaningful pictures, poems, quotations, notes, or just a few words may provide the opportunity to abstract meaning from the experience of living with a communication disorder (Pound et al., 2000).

Therapeutic writing or journaling may also offer benefits to the families and support persons of those with communication disorders. Those living with communication disorder, including family members, support persons, and friends, need to make meaning from the events that they have experienced. Their coping strategies and adjustment could be facilitated by participating in a therapeutic writing paradigm, such as the 30-minute daily writing sessions for three to five times. Journaling has often been used and reported as providing an outlet for positive and negative emotions, and as a way to actively reflect on events as they transpire.

For example, Schwartz and Drotar (2004) employed this therapeutic writing paradigm with caregivers of children with chronic illnesses. Two groups of caregivers were compared. Twenty-nine caregivers in the experimental group wrote for 20 minutes about traumatic experiences on 3 different days, while the control group of 24 caregivers wrote about summer activities on 3 different days. Baseline measures of physical health-related quality of life were taken and compared to performance on the same measures 4 months later. Cognition- and emotion-related words were analyzed across the three writing sample times. Caregivers in the experimental group who wrote about traumatic experiences used more emotion and cognition words than the control group. A decrease in negative emotion words and an increase in the use of cognition words were linked to better physical health quality of life. This project suggests that a therapeutic writing paradigm may produce important benefits to caregivers of children with chronic illnesses or disabilities. A similar outcome might also result for caregivers and support persons of adults living with chronic disability, including communication disabilities.

Speech-language pathologists should consider actively employing these tools to facilitate improvement in coping and adjustment to living with communication disorders. Most importantly, the measurement of a broad range of clinical outcomes should be employed and intervention comparisons made to determine whether these activities provide benefit and if so, what kind of benefit can reasonably be expected.

Therapeutic letter writing has been used as an effective tool, particularly in family therapy when families are separated by distance or by understanding (Davidson & Birmingham, 2001). In this activity, an individual writes a letter to one or more family members, and other members of the family write letters in turn. This procedure can be used to facilitate actual communication or as an exercise to evolve reactions and responses to family members. Speech-language pathologists could be in the position of helping clients write to family members or friends about how they feel about communication patterns in the family, or how they feel communication strategies could be improved to facilitate effective communication. In some cases, I have known of individuals with communication disorders to write letters to the editor of the local paper to share tips and strategies that will facilitate communication.

Developing a narrative about one's own disability both reflects current coping state and facilitates the development of coping. One way in which this has commonly been done in speech-language pathology is through the development of support groups. The canonical illness story that may be generated in a support group setting serves as a way for individuals to gather a sense of meaning and shared experience. It also provides a means for individuals to consider how their own set of circumstances is both similar to and different from others with the same condition. It would be interesting for speech-language pathologists to explore the general narratives that are produced in support group settings, as well as the individual stories that come from the social context of shared experience.

Narrative forms not only facilitate coping strategies with concomitant physical and psychological health benefits, but also may decrease the level of stress experienced by those adjusting to the onset of communication disorder. It may be that certain aspects of stories about living with a communication disorder could be more beneficial at certain points along the adjustment continuum. Understanding the relationships between self-produced narratives, hearing the narratives of others in similar circumstances, and the patterns of coping and adjustment could better arm speech-language pathologists to facilitate psychosocial adjustment in persons living with communication disorders.

Bibliotherapy

Bibliotherapy and poetry therapy are techniques that have been little discussed in speech-language pathology, although the general principle may have likely been used by some clinicians informally. In these cases, books or poetry with healing and positive themes are employed to facilitate discussion, reaction, and positive response (McArdle & Byrt, 2001). Poetry and literature in therapy facilitate greater self-understanding and self-esteem, expressing overwhelming emotions and releasing stress, and improving coping skills (Gorelick, 2005). It would seem that support groups might be a likely context in which to discuss particular stories or poems about living with a disability or otherwise overcoming adversity. We have many poems that have been written by those living with communication disorders, as well as books about their personal experience, and these could serve as potential targets. For adult language disorders, book clubs have been used as a format to facilitate improvement in reading comprehension and specifically reading for pleasure (Elman et al., 2004; Elman et al., 2005). In this format, it might be interesting to select, with the group members, a book that offers a positive healing theme or message.

Bibliotherapy has been defined as the interaction between the reader and the text (Silverberg, 2003). Just as in a clinician-client relationship, a dynamic develops between a reader and the literature that can include projection of one's self into the text and the development of insight and introspection. Texts are chosen that can enhance discussion and reflection of problems and dilemmas similar to the readers. The emotional processes, which are fundamental to bibliotherapy, include identification, catharsis, and the development of insight (Sridhar & Vaughn, 2002). The potential outcomes of a bibliotherapy intervention can be cognitive or informational, behavioral in terms of changing behaviors, and/or emotional and interactional.

Two types of texts have been described as appropriate for bibliotherapy (Silverberg, 2003). Didactic texts have often been used to present conceptual and procedural information to patients about a diagnosis or a desired behavior change. Literary texts are also potentially strong sources for bibliotherapy, and might engage the reader in the story and the dilemma of the characters in a meaningful and constructive way.

Sufficient study has been conducted in some areas that employ bibliotherapy to produce a meta-analysis (Apodaca & Miller, 2003). A meta-analysis of 22 studies investigated the use of self-help materials on changing drinking behavior. Moderate support was found for the use of bibliotherapy in the form of self-help materials for problem drinkers who self-identified and were seeking help to change their drinking behaviors.

Bibliotherapy has also been employed with individuals with learning disabilities. A meta-analysis suggested a modest but important association between bibliotherapy and the improvement of self-concept among students with various learning disabilities (Sridhar & Vaughn, 2002). The approach also has been linked to both improved self-concept and improved reading comprehension for students learning English as a second language.

A typical bibliotherapy approach employs the activation of previous knowledge prior to learning by reviewing related concepts or settings of those linked to the targeted text (Sridhar & Vaughan, 2002). During and after reading, students and teachers generate questions, comment, and paraphrase and reflect on the meaning of the text to themselves or to their own experiences. This provides the necessary opportunity to identify with the characters in the text and to emotionally process the issues raised by the reading.

Bibliotherapy has been shown to produce positive results in well-being and self-management ability among 97 older adults who were mildly to moderately frail, compared to 96 older adults who participated in a delayed-treatment control condition (Frieswijk, Steverink, Buunk, & Slaets, 2005). Self-management ability was defined as the ability to obtain resources necessary to compensate for physical and psychosocial losses, associated with the aging process. In this study, the inexpensive bibliotherapy intervention facilitated teaching older adults how to cull desirable resources.

Bibliotherapy has also been shown to be a powerful treatment choice for treating depression in older adults. For example, a direct comparison between individual cognitive psychotherapy with bibliotherapy (reading the book *Feeling Good* by Bums, 1980) produced significantly positive outcomes of both treatments compared to a delayed-treatment control condition (Floyd, Scogin, McKendree-Smith, Floyd, & Rokke, 2004). Self-reported ratings of depression were higher for individual psychotherapy, but clinician ratings of depression outcomes were similar for both the individual psychotherapy and the bibliotherapy.

In a study of the preferences of patients with head and neck cancer, patients indicated a preference for individual, one-on-one cognitive-behavioral therapy for psychological issues resulting from the cancer (Semple, Dunwoody, Sullivan, & Kernohan, 2006). This preference was followed closely by bibliotherapy, and the last choice of patients was for group therapy.

Summary

Many intervention approaches and techniques that are currently in existence and in use in speech-language pathology are likely to offer positive benefits to the client in terms of development of a sense of self, facilitating compliance and adherence to a new regimen, reducing stress, and increasing coping. As clinicians we may often select certain therapeutic procedures precisely because we feel that a particular client would benefit in one or more of these ways from the selected intervention. We do not always acknowledge these benefits formally by documenting changes in these areas or by researching potential changes associated with particular treatments. A narrative-based approach emphasizes the story of the client—the story of his life and his illness/disability. It can broaden the scope of clinical tools already in use and lead to the innovation of new techniques that can holistically address the communication needs of our clients.

STUDY/DISCUSSION QUESTIONS AND ACTIVITIES

1. Describe one way in which you already use personal narrative in intervention and discuss potential outcomes that you have not previously measured or explored.
2. Consider one new way in which you might incorporate personal narrative into your clinical activities.

APPENDIX
1

Summary of Guidelines and Requirements for Earning ASHA CEUs

Always consult the American Speech-Language-Hearing Association (ASHA) Web site (http://www.asha.org) to ensure that policies and procedures are current. Learning Objectives and Study/Discussion Questions and Activities are provided throughout the book to provide examples for learning activities.

There are two ways for professionals to earn Continuing Education Units (CEUs) from ASHA through study that includes the use of this book. One way is to use the book or portions of the book in an independent study plan. A second way is to use the book as part of a journal study group.

1. Independent Study Plan for ASHA CEUs

An independent study is a self-designed set of learning activities that contribute to a professional's growth in a particular topic area. To earn ASHA CEUs for an independent study activity, you must follow the procedures and complete the forms available on the ASHA Web site. Your independent study will be reviewed, evaluated, and monitored by an independent study sponsor who is an ASHA approved CE sponsor. On the required ASHA form, you will need to provide a title and description of the activity, and indicate the dates of the activity. You must identify a subject code for the independent study. If you are using this book as some part of an independent study, you may find that Subject Codes 7010 (Service Delivery) and 7020 (Education and Training) are the best fits for your activity. You may also find that the topics addressed in this book are most consistent with the Professional content area.

You will need to identify your own personal learning objectives for your independent study—these are not to be the objectives of the course material or an instructor. So, you may consider the Learning Objectives offered at the beginning of each chapter in this book as examples that will help you formulate your own learning objectives. Similarly, the Study/Discussion Questions and Activities at the end of each chapter may also help you to identify useful outcome activities and/or assessments that you might incorporate into an independent study. Of course, the purpose of the independent study is self-development of learning, so you should think about your own practice and professional interests as you develop your objectives and measures.

2. Journal Study Groups

Form a journal study group with from 4 to 10 other professionals. Follow the instructions on the ASHA Web site and download the forms you will need to register your group and identify your group members. You will also need to identify a coordinator for the group. ASHA procedures for journal study groups require that you complete forms identifying topics and learning objectives and that attendance records be maintained over the course of the group's meetings.

ASHA provides a list of journals that can serve as sources for a journal study group. Check with ASHA first to ensure that material from this book or any other will be acceptable sources for earning ASHA CEUs through a journal study group. You might want to design a combination or series of readings that include some book material with related journal articles, for example. In every case, however, be sure to plan your study group and get approval from ASHA *first* before carrying out your plan.

APPENDIX
2

Sociocultural Issues in Narrative

The following is an initial bibliography on the topic of sociocultural variations in narrative. Although the structure and sequence of narrative forms is not a primary topic in this book, it is important to understand the differences in narrative forms as they relate to different cultural perspectives. This brief bibliography on the topic of cultural issues and narrative form is offered as a starting point for those interested in pursuing this topic further.

Bedore, L. M., Fiestas, C. E., Peña, E. D., & Nagy, V. J. (2006). Cross-language comparison of maze use in Spanish and English in functionally monolingual and bilingual children. *Bilingualism: Language & Cognition, 9,* 233-247.

Daiute, C., & Lightfoot, C. (Eds.). (2004). *Narrative analysis: Studying the development of individuals in society.* Thousand Oaks, CA: Sage.

Ghosh, A. K. (2004). Doctor-patient communication: Emerging challenges. *Family Practice, 21,* 114-115.

Kang, J. Y. (2004). Telling a coherent story in a foreign language: Analysis of Korean EFL learners' referential strategies in oral narrative discourse. *Journal of Pragmatics, 36,* 1975-1990.

Li, W. (2004). Topic chains in Chinese discourse. *Discourse Processes, 37,* 25-45.

Luchjenbroers, J. (Ed.) *Cognitive linguistics investigations*. Amsterdam: John Benjamins.

Majors, Y. J. (2004). "I wasn't scared of them, they were scared of me": Constructions of self/other in a Midwestern hair salon. *Anthropology & Education Quarterly, 35*, 167–188.

Morgan, G. (2006). The development of narrative skills in British Sign Language. In B. Schick, M. Marschak, & P. E. Spencer (Eds.), *Advances in the sign language development of deaf children*. New York: Oxford University Press.

Morgan, M. (2004). Signifying laughter and the subtleties of loud-talking: Memory and meaning in African-American women's discourse. In M. Farr (Ed.), *Ethnolinguistic Chicago: Language and literacy in the city's neighborhoods*. Mahwah, NJ: Lawrence Erlbaum.

Moss, B., & Roberts, C. (2005). Explanations, explanations, explanations: How do patients with limited English construct narrative accounts in multilingual, multiethnic settings, and how can GPs interpret them? *Family Practice, 22*, 412–418.

Ohtaki, S., Ohtaki, T., & Fetters, M. D. (2003). Doctor-patient communication: A comparison of the USA and Japan. *Family Practice, 20*, 276–282.

Phillion, J., Fang He, M., & Connelly, F. M. (Eds.). (2005). *Narrative & experience in multicultural education*. Thousand Oaks, CA: Sage.

Ramirez-Esparza, N., & Pennebaker, J. W. (2006). Do good stories produce good health? Exploring words, language, and culture. *Narrative Inquiry, 16*, 211–219.

Robinson, T. L., & Crowe, T. A. (1998). Culture-based considerations in programming for stuttering intervention with African American clients and their families. *Language, Speech, and Hearing Services in Schools, 29*, 172–179.

Stromqvist, S., & Verhoeven, L. (Eds.). (2004). *Relating events in narrative: Vol. 2. Typological and contextual perspectives*. Mahwah, NJ: Lawrence Erlbaum Associates.

Ulatowska, H. K., Olness, G. S., Samson, A. M., Keebler, M. W., & Goins, K. W. (2004). On the nature of personal narratives of high quality. *Advances in Speech-Language Pathology, 6*, 3–14.

Verhoeven, L., & Stromquist, S. (Eds.). (2001). *Narrative development in a multilingual context*. Philadelphia: J. Benjamin.

APPENDIX
3

Personal Narratives of People Living with Communication Disorders

The following is a list of published personal narratives of individuals living with communication disorders. The list is grouped by general communication disability category for convenience. Unfortunately, this list cannot be comprehensive since new narratives are constantly being published, often self-published and marketed through the Internet. This list is a good starting point for those interested in reading published stories about living with a communication disorder.

For most of my career, I have kept a file of newspaper clips, magazine articles, and books that have been authored by people living with aphasia, my own practice specialty. I imagine that many other clinicians have done the same thing, and have their own sources of this type to reflect on and share. The following list of published books has been useful to me in teaching various courses; I have almost always tried to bring the voice of the people we are learning to serve into each of my courses by requiring the reading of at least one personal narrative relevant to the course.

Published narratives of those living with communication disorders can also serve as a resource for clients, families, and friends who are learning to cope with a communication disorder. Sharing narratives of others living with a similar communication disability needs to be done with care, of course. Reading such an account can bring forward dangerous emotions that an individual may not yet be ready to deal with if such a thing is done without caution. Some narratives may raise issues, worries, and fears that readers had not yet thought of, adding to their care burden. Each clinician must use careful judgment, as always, when suggesting these materials to those affected by the disorder. My approach is to let people know that these books are in existence, that there are many others out there who are living in similar situations. Then I wait to see if the individual initiates an interest in knowing more about the published accounts. In my view, published accounts present more of a risk to an individual's psychic state, potentially, then a support group or other immediate social interaction, where similar narratives might also be offered. In a support group, when the interaction is live, questions can be asked, clarifications made, hugs, smiles, and Kleenex offered in a supportive environment. Books can do none of those things. Reading a published account alone may exacerbate a sense of isolation and desperation. As in all of our clinical activities, we must use an educated and heightened sensitivity to the potential psychological impact of our actions.

About Personal Narratives/Disability Narratives

Ryan, E. B. (2006). Finding a new voice: Writing through health adversity. *Journal of Language and Social Psychology, 22,* 423–436.

Acquired Language-Cognitive Disorders (cognitive-linguistic impairment due to TBI; aphasia; right hemisphere disorder)

Adamson, K. (2002). *Kate's journey: Triumph over adversity.* Retrieved from http://www.katesjourney.com

Albertson, E. T. (1947). A glimpse into an aphasic's world. *American Journal of Occupational Therapy, 1,* 361-364.

Alexander, E. (1990, Summer). Aphasia—The worm's eye view of a philosophic patient and the medical establishment. *Diogenes, 150,* 1-23.

Berger, P., & Mensch, S. (1999). *How to conquer the world with one hand . . . and an attitude.* Merillat, VA: Positive Power.

Bryant, B. (1992). *In search of wings: A journey back from traumatic brain injury.* San Antonio: Wings Publishing.

Buck, M. (1963). The language disorders: A personal and professional account of aphasia. *Journal of Rehabilitation, 29,* 37-38.

Caplan, L. R., & Hutton, C. (2003). *Striking back at stroke: A doctor-patient journal.* Washington, DC: Dana Press.

Crimmins, C. (2001). *Where is the mango princess?* London: Vintage.

Critchley, M. (1962). Dr. Samuel Johnson's aphasia. *Medical History, 6,* 27-46.

Cuddihy, R. G. (2000). *Merry-go-sorry, a memoir of joy and sadness.* Albuquerque, NM: Cuddihy Enterprises.

Dahlberg, C. C., & Jaffe, J. J. (1977). *Stroke: A doctor's personal story of his recovery.* New York: W. W. Norton.

Ewing, S. A., & Pfalzgraf, B. (1991). *Pathways: Moving beyond stroke and aphasia.* Detroit, MI: Wayne State University Press.

Farrell, B. (1969). *Pat and Roald: The story of Patricia Neal's stroke and recovery.* New York: Random House.

Hall, W. A. (1961). Return from silence: A personal experience. *Journal of Speech and Hearing Disorders, 26,* 174-176.

Hinds, D. M., & Morris, P. (2000). *After stroke.* New York: Thorsons.

Hodgins, E. (1964). *Episode: Report on the accident inside my skull.* New York: Atheneum.

Hoff, H. E., Guillemin, R., & Geddes, L. A. (1958). An 18th century scientist's observations of his own aphasia. *Bulletin of Historical Medicine, 32,* 446-450.

Hughes, K. (1990). *God isn't finished with me yet.* Nashville, TN: Winston-Derek.

Josephs, A. (1992). *The invaluable guide to life after stroke: An owner's manual.* Long Beach, CA: Amadeus Press.

Kapur, N. (Ed.). (1997). *Injured brains of medical minds: Views from within.* New York: Oxford University Press.

Kemp, B. J., & Mosqueda, L. (2004). *Aging with a disability: What the clinician needs to know.* Baltimore: Johns Hopkins University Press.

Knox, D. (1985). *Portrait of aphasia.* Detroit, MI: Wayne State University Press.

Krupnick, S. (1986). *Stroke! The ordeal and the rainbow.* Gerald, MO: The Patrice Press.

Lavin, J. H. (1985). *Stroke: From crisis to victory—A family guide*. New York: Franklin Watts.

Luria, A. R. (1968). *The mind of a mnemonist: A little book about a vast memory*. Jackson, TN: Basic Books.

Luria, A. R. (2004). *The man with a shattered world: The history of a brain wound*. Cambridge, MA: Harvard University Press.

Luterman, D. (1995). *In the shadows: Living and coping with a loved one's chronic illness*. Bedford, MA: Jade Press.

Martin, V. (1997). *Out of my head: An experience with neurosurgery*. Philadelphia: Trans-Atlantic.

Matthewson, M. (1997). *Courage after coma: A family's journey*. Alberta: Uneek Experience.

McBride, C. (1969). *Silent victory*. Chicago: Nelson Hall.

McCrum, R. (1999). *My year off: Recovering life after a stroke*. New York: Broadway.

Mills, H. (2004). *A mind of my own: Memoir of recovery from aphasia*. Authorhouse.

Moss, S. (1972). *Recovery with aphasia: The aftermath of my stroke*. Chicago: University of Illinois Press.

Newborn, B. (1997). *Return to Ithaca*. Bergenfield, NJ: Penguin USA.

Osborn, C. L. (2000). *Over my head: A doctor's own story of head injury from the inside looking out*. Riverside, NJ: Andrews McMeel.

Parr, S., Byng, S., & Gilpin, S. (with Ireland, C.). (1997). *Talking about aphasia*. Philadelphia: Open University Press.

Perez, P. (2001). *Brain attack: Danger, chaos, opportunity, and empowerment*. Johnson, VT: Cutting Edge Press.

Porus, S. (2003). *Is that really me?* Retrieved from http://www.shirley porus.com

Quann, E. S. (2002). *By his side—Life and love after stroke*. Highland, MD: Fastrak Press.

Quinn, D. A. (1998). *Conquering the darkness: One woman's story of recovering from a brain injury*. St. Paul, MN: Paragon House.

Riese, W. (1954). Auto-observation reported by eminent nineteenth century medical scientist. *Bulletin of Historical Medicine, 28*, 237–242.

Ritchie, D. (1966). *Stroke: A diary of recovery*. London: Faber and Faber.

Rolnick, M., & Hoops, H. R. (1970). Aphasia as seen by the aphasic. *Journal of Speech and Hearing Disorders, 34*, 48–53.

Rose, R. H. (1948). A physician's account of his own aphasia. *Journal of Speech and Hearing Disorders, 13*, 294–305.

Ruth, B. (1995). *November days: A love story*. Denver, CO: Frances Scott Press.

Sies, L. F., & Butler, B. (1963). A personal account of dysphasia. *Journal of Speech and Hearing Disorders, 28*, 261–266.

Smith, R. F. (2005). *Stroke of midnight: A brain attack.* Retrieved from http://www.thestrokeofmidnight.com

Sorrell, M. (1969). *Out of silence.* UK: Stoughton Limited.

Swanson, K. K. (1999). *I'll carry the fork!* Scotts Valley, CA: Rising Star Press.

Wender, D. (1986 , March 25). At the edge of silence. *Family Circle,* 62–69.

Wender, D. (1987). "Craziness" and "visions": Experiences after a stroke. *British Medical Journal, 295,* 1595–1597.

Wender, D. (1989). Aphasic victim as investigator. *Archives of Neurology, 46,* 91–92.

Wint, G. (1967). *The third killer.* New York: Abelard-Schuman.

Wulf, H. (1974; 1986). *Aphasia, my world alone.* Detroit, MI: Wayne State University Press.

Living with Dementia

Chene, B. (2006). Dementia and residential placement: A view from the carer's perspective. *Qualitative Social Work: Research and Practice, 5,* 187–215.

Harman, G., & Clare, L. (2006). Illness representations and lived experience in early-stage dementia. *Qualitative Health Research, 16,* 484–502.

Page, S., & Fletcher, T. (2006). Auguste D. *The International Journal of Social Research and Practice, 5,* 571–583.

Swensen, C. R. (2004). Dementia diary: A personal and professional journal. *Social Work, 49,* 451–460.

General Illness: Children

Forsner, M., Janssen, L., & Soerlie, V. (2005). Being ill as narrated by children aged 11–18 years. *Journal of Child Health Care, 9,* 314–323.

Language and Learning Disabilities

Cordoni, B. (1990). *Living with a learning disability.* Carbondale: Southern Illinois University Press.

Dillon, K. M. (1995). *Living with autism: The parents' stories.* Boone, NC: Parkway.

Hallowell, E. M., & Ratey, J. (1994). *Driven to distraction.* New York: Simon & Schuster.

Handler, L. (2004). *Twitch and shout: A Touretter's tale.* Minneapolis: University of Minnesota Press.

Hughes, S. (1990). *Ryan—A mother's story of her hyperactive/Tourette syndrome child.* Duarte, CA: Hope Press.

Kennedy, M. A. (2001). *My perfect son has cerebral palsy: A mother's guide of helpful hints.* Bloomington, IN: Authorhouse.

Klein, S. D., & Schive, K. (2006). *You will dream new dreams: Inspiring personal stories by parents of children with disabilities.* New York: Kensington.

Osman, B. B. (1997). *Learning disabilities and ADHD: A family guide to living and learning together.* Hoboken, NJ: Wiley.

Riddick, B. (1996). *Living with dyslexia: The social and emotional consequences of specific learning difficulties.* Oxford, UK: Routeledge.

Rubio, G. H. (2001). *Icy sparks.* London: Penguin.

Willey, L. H. (1999). *Pretending to be normal: Living with Asperger's syndrome.* Philadelphia: Kingsley.

Fluency

Carlisle, J. A. (1986). *Tangled tongue.* Boston: Addison Wesley.

St. Louis, K. O. (2001). *Living with stuttering.* Morgantown, WV: Populore.

Motor Speech Disorders

Douglas, K. (2002). *My stroke of luck.* New York: Harper Collins.

Hollins, S., Barnett, S., & Redmond, D. (1997). *Michelle finds a voice.* London: Gaskell/St. George's Hospital Medical School.

References

Abma, T. A., & Widdershoven, G. A. M. (2005). Sharing stories: Narrative and dialogue in responsive nursing evaluation. *Evaluation and the Health Professions, 28*, 90-108.

Adams, C., Lloyd, J., & Aldred, C. (2006). Exploring the effects of communication intervention for developmental pragmatic language impairments: A signal-generation study. *International Journal of Language & Communication Disorders, 41*, 41-65.

Affleck, G., & Tennen, H. (1996). Construing benefits from adversity: Adaptational significance and dispositional underpinnings. *Journal of Personality, 64*, 899-922.

Aita, V., McIlwain, H., Backer, E., McVea, K., & Crabtree, B. (2005). Patient-centered care and communication in primary care practice: What is involved? *Patient Education and Counseling*, [Special issue]. *Medical Education and Training in Communication, 58*, 296-304.

Albertson, E. T. (1947). A glimpse into an aphasic's world. *American Journal of Occupational Therapy, 1*, 361-364.

Allman, J. L. (1996). Bearing the burden or baring the soul: Physicians' self-disclosure and boundary management regarding medical mistakes. *Dissertation Abstracts International, 56(8A)*, 2935.

American Speech-Language-Hearing Association. (2004). *Evidence-Based Practice in Communication Disorders: An Introduction* [Technical Report]. Available from www.asha.org/policy

American Speech-Language-Hearing Association. (2005). *Evidence-Based Practice in Communication Disorders* [Position Statement]. Available from www.asha.org/policy

Ames, S. C., Patten, C. A., & Offord, K. P. (2005). Expressive writing intervention for young adult cigarette smokers. *Journal of Clinical Psychology, 61*, 1555–1570.

Anderson, H., & Goolishian, H. (1992). The client is the expert: A not-knowing approach to therapy. In S. McNamee & K. J. Gergen (Eds.), *Therapy as social construction* (pp. 25–39). Newbury Park, CA: Sage.

Anderson, S., & Marlett, N. J. (2004). The language of recovery: How effective communication of information is crucial to restructuring post-stroke life. *Topics in Stroke Rehabilitation, 11*, 55–67.

Angrosino, M. V. (1998). *Opportunity house: Ethnographic stories of mental retardation.* Walnut Creek, CA: AltaMira Press.

Apodaca, T. R., & Miller, W. R. (2003). A meta-analysis of the effectiveness of bibliotherapy for alcohol problems. *Journal of Clinical Psychology, 59*, 289–304.

Arts, J. A. R., Gijselaers, W. H., & Segers, M. S. R. (2006). Enhancing problem-solving expertise by means of an authentic, collaborative, computer supported and problem-based course. *European Journal of Psychology of Education, 21*, 71–90.

Baltes, P. B. (2003). On the incomplete architecture of human ontogeny: Selection, optimization and compensation as foundation of developmental theory. In U. M. Staudinger & U. Lindenberger (Eds.), *Understanding human development: Dialogues with lifespan psychology.* Dordrecht, Netherlands: Kluwer Academic Publishers.

Barnard, M. (2005). Discomforting research: Colliding moralities and looking for "truth" in a study of parental drug problems. *Sociology of Health & Illness, 27*, 1–19.

Barnato, A. E., Labor, R. E., Freeborne, N. E., Jayes, R. L., Campbell, D. E., & Lynn, J. (2005). Qualitative analysis of Medicare claims in the last three years of life: A pilot study. *Journal of the American Geriatrics Society, 53*, 66–72.

Barrett, M. S., & Berman, J. S. (2001). Is psychotherapy more effective when therapists disclose personal information about themselves? *Journal of Consulting and Clinical Psychology, 69*, 597–603.

Barrows, A. R. (2004). *Narratives of stroke and aphasia: An ethnographic investigation.* Unpublished doctoral dissertation, Trinity College, Dublin, Ireland.

Bateson, M. C. (1989). *Composing a life.* New York: Atlantic Monthly Press.

Beach, M. C., Roter, D., Larson, S., Levinson, W., Ford, D. E., & Frankel, R. (2004). What do physicians tell patients about themselves? A qualitative analysis of physician self-disclosure. *Journal of General Internal Medicine, 19*, 911–916.

Beach, W. A. & Mandelbaum, J. (2005). "My Mom had a stroke": Understanding how patients raise and providers respond to psychosocial concerns. In L. M. Harter, P. M. Japp, & C. S. Beck (Eds.), *Narratives, health, and healing: Communication theory, research, and practice.* Mahwah, NJ: Lawrence Erlbaum Associates.

Beck, C. S. (2005). Becoming the story: Narratives as collaborative, social enactments of individual, relational, and public identities. In L. M. Harter, P. M. Japp, & C. S. Beck (Eds.), *Narratives, health, and healing: Communication theory, research, and practice.* Mahwah, NJ: Lawrence Erlbaum Associates.

Beckwith, K. M. (2003). The effects of expressive writing on blood pressure, psychosocial adjustment, and heart rate variability in high normal to moderate high blood pressure. *Dissertation Abstracts International, 64*(2-B), 995.

Behar, R. (1997). *The vulnerable observer: Anthropology that breaks your heart.* Boston: Beacon.

Belzen, J. A. (1996). Beyond a classic? Hjalmar Sunden's role theory and contemporary narrative psychology. *International Journal for the Psychology of Religion, 6*, 181–199.

Bennett-Levy, J. (2006). Therapist skills: A cognitive model of their acquisition and refinement. *Behavioural and Cognitive Psychotherapy, 34*, 57–78.

Berg, G. A. (2000). Cognitive development through narrative: Computer interface design for educational purposes. *Journal of Educational Multimedia and Hypermedia, 9*, 3–17.

Berman, J. (2001). Teaching students at risk. *PsyART, 5*, Article 010131. Retrieved June 11, 2007, from http://www.clas.ufl.edu/ipsa/journal/2001_berman01.shtml

Bettelheim, B. (1976). *The uses of enchantment.* New York: Alfred A. Knopf.

Biddle, K. R., McCabe, A., & Bliss, L. (1996). Narrative skills following traumatic brain injury in children and adults. *Journal of Communication Disorders, 29*, 447–469.

Bleakley, A. (2005). Stories as data, data as stories: Making sense of narrative inquiry in clinical education. *Medical Education, 39*, 534–540.

Bliss, L. S., McCabe, A., & Miranda, A. E. (1998). Narrative assessment profile: Discourse analysis for school-age children. *Journal of Communication Disorders, 31*, 347–363.

Bloom, R. L. (1994). Hemispheric responsibility and discourse production: Contrasting patients with unilateral left and right hemisphere damage. In R. Bloom, L. K. Obler, S. DeSanti, & J. S. Ehrlich (Eds.), *Discourse analysis and applications: Studies in adult clinical populations.* Hillsdale, NJ: Erlbaum.

Bolton, G. (2005). Medicine and literature: Writing and reading. *Journal of Evaluation in Clinical Practice, 11*, 171–179.

Brandell, J. R., & Varkas, T. (2001). Narrative case studies. In B. A. Thyer (Ed.), *The handbook of social work research methods.* Thousand Oaks, CA: Sage.

Brewer, W. F. (1986). What is autobiographical memory? In D. Rubin (Ed.), *Autobiographical memory.* New York: Cambridge University Press.

Brinton, B., & Fujiki, M. (2002). Social development in children with specific language impairment and profound hearing loss. In P. K. Smith & C. H. Hart (Eds.), *Blackwell handbook of childhood social development.* Malden, MA: Blackwell.

Brinton, B., Fujiki, M., & Highee, L. (1998). Participation in cooperative learning activities by children with specific language impairment. *Journal of Speech, Language, & Hearing Research, 41,* 1193–1206.

Brinton, B., Robinson, L. A., & Fujiki, M. (2004). Description of a program for social language intervention: "If you can have a conversation, you can have a relationship." *Language, Speech, and Hearing Services in Schools, 35,* 283–290.

Brockmeier, J., & Carbaugh, D. (2001). Introduction. In J. Brockmeier & D. Carbaugh (Eds.), *Narrative and identity: Studies in autobiography, self and culture.* Philadelphia: John Benjamins.

Brockmeier, J., & Harre, R. (2001). Narrative: Problems and promises of an alternative paradigm. In J. Brockmeier & D. Carbaugh (Eds.), *Narrative and identity: Studies in autobiography, self and culture.* Philadelphia: John Benjamins.

Brownell, H., & Martino, G. (1998). Deficits in inference and social cognition: The effects of right hemisphere brain damage on discourse. In M. Beesman & C. Chiarello (Eds.), *Right hemisphere language comprehension: Perspectives from cognitive neuroscience.* Hillsdale, NJ: Erlbaum.

Bruner, J. (1986). *Actual minds, possible worlds.* Cambridge, MA: Harvard University Press.

Bruner, J. S. (1990). *Acts of meaning.* Cambridge, MA: Harvard University Press.

Bruner, J. (2001). Self-making and world-making. In J. Brockmeier & D. Carbaugh (Eds.), *Narrative and identity: Studies in autobiography, self and culture.* Philadelphia: John Benjamins.

Bruner, J. (2003). Self-making narratives. In R. Fivush & C. A. Haden (Eds.), *Autobiographical memory and the construction of a narrative self: Developmental and cultural perspectives.* Mahwah, NJ: Lawrence Erlbaum.

Bulow, P. H. (2004). Sharing experiences of contested illness by storytelling. *Discourse & Society, 15*(1), 33–53.

Byrne, B. (2003). Reciting the self: Narrative representations of the self in qualitative interviews. *Feminist Theory, 4,* 29–49.

Caplan, S. E., Haslett, B. J., & Burleson, B. R. (2005). Telling it like it is: The adaptive function of narratives in coping with loss in later life. *Health Communication, 17,* 233–251.

Carbaugh, D. A. (1996). *Situating selves: The communication of social identities in American scenes.* Albany, NY: State University of New York Press.

Casey, B., & Long, A. (2002). Reconciling voices. *Journal of Psychiatric and Mental Health Nursing, 9*(5), 603–610.

Caspari, I., & Parkinson, S. R. (2000). Effects of memory impairment on discourse. *Journal of Neurolinguistics, 13,* 15–36.

Cercle, A. (2002). Textual and narratological analysis of the social representation of alcoholism in a self-help group. *European Review of Applied Psychology/Revue Européenne de Psychologie Appliquée, 52,* 253–261.

Chan, E. A., Cheung, K., Mok, E., Cheung, S., & Tong, E. (2006). A narrative inquiry into the Hong Kong Chinese adults' concepts of health through their cultural stories. *International Journal of Nursing Studies, 43,* 301–309.

Chandler, G. E., (2002). An evaluation of college and low-income youth writing together: Self-discovery and cultural connection. *Issues in Comprehensive Pediatric Nursing, 25,* 255–269.

Chapman, S. B., Highley, A. P. & Thompson, J. L. (1998). Discourse in fluent aphasia and Alzheimer's disease: Linguistic and pragmatic considerations. *Journal of Neurolinguistics, 11,* 55–78.

Chelf, J. H., Deshler, A. M. B., Hillman, S., & Durazo-Arvizu, R. (2000). Storytelling: A strategy for living and coping with cancer. *Cancer Nursing, 23,* 1–5.

Cherney, L. R. (1998). Pragmatics and discourse: An introduction. In L. R. Cherney, B. B. Shadden, & C. A. Coelho (Eds.), *Analyzing discourse in communicatively impaired adults.* Gaithersburg, MD: Aspen.

Cherney, L. R., & Canter, G. J. (1993). Informational content in the discourse of patients with probable Alzheimer's disease and patients with right brain damage. In M. Lemme (Ed.), *Clinical aphasiology* (Vol. 2). Austin, TX: Pro-Ed.

Cherney, L. R., Drimmer, D. P., & Halper, A. S. (1997). Informational content and unilateral neglect: A longitudinal investigation of five subjects with right hemisphere damage. *Aphasiology, 11,* 351–363.

Chi, M., Glaser, R., & Farr, M. (Eds.). (1988). *The nature of expertise.* Mahwah, New Jersey: Lawrence Erlbaum.

Clandinin, J., & Connelly, M. (2000). *Narrative inquiry: Experience and story in qualitative research.* San Francisco: Jossy-Bass.

Clark, M. M. (2005). Holocaust video testimony, oral history, and narrative medicine: The struggle against indifference. *Literature and Medicine, 24,* 266–282.

Cocude, M., Mellet, E., & Denis, M. (1999). Visual and mental exploration of visual-spatial configurations: Behavioral and neuroimaging approaches. *Psychological Research, 62*, 93–106.

Coelho, C. A. (2002). Story narratives of adults with closed head injury and non-brain-injured adults: Influence of socioeconomic status, elicitation task, and executive functioning. *Journal of Speech, Language, & Hearing Research, 45*, 1232–1249.

Coelho, C. A., Grela, B., Corso, M., Gamble, A., & Feinn, R. (2005). Microlinguistic deficits in the narrative discourse of adults with traumatic brain injury. *Brain Injury, 19*, 1139–1145.

Cohler, B. J. (1982). Personal narrative and the life course. In P. Baltes & O. G. Brin, Jr. (Eds.), *Life span development and behavior* (Vol. 4). New York: Academic Press.

Conway, M. A., & Pleydell-Pearce, C. W. (2000). The construction of autobiographical memories in the self-memory system. *Psychological Review, 107*, 261–288.

Cortazzi, M., Jin, L., Wall, D., & Cavendish, S. (2001). Sharing learning through narrative communication. *International Journal of Language & Communication Disorders, 36*, 252–257.

Craig, H. K., & Washington, J. A. (1993). The access behaviors of children with specific language impairment. *Journal of Speech and Hearing Research, 36*, 322–337.

Crane, S. L., & Cooper, E. B. (1983). Speech-language clinician personality variables and clinical effectiveness. *Journal of Speech and Hearing Disorders, 48*, 140–145.

Cross, M. (1999). Lost for words. *Child and Family Social Work, 4*, 249–257.

Crossley, M. L. (2000). Narrative psychology, trauma and the study of self/identity. *Theory & Psychology, 10*(4), 527–546.

Crossley, M. L. (2003). Formulating narrative psychology: The limitations of contemporary social constructionism. *Narrative Inquiry, 13*, 287–300.

Damico, J. S., & Simmons-Mackie, N. N. (2003). Qualitative research and speech-language pathology: A tutorial for the clinical realm. *American Journal of Speech-Language Pathology, 12*, 131–143.

Damico, J. S., Simmons-Mackie, N., Oelschlaeger, M., Elman, R., & Armstrong, E. (1999). Qualitative methods in aphasia research: Basic issues. *Aphasiology, 13*, 651–665.

DasGupta, S., & Charon, R. (2004). Personal illness narratives: Using reflective writing to teach empathy. *Academic Medicine, 79*, 351–356.

DasGupta, S., Meyer, D., Calero-Breckheimer, A., Costley, A. W., & Guillen, S. (2006). Teaching cultural competency through narrative medicine: Intersections of classroom and community. *Teaching and Learning in Medicine, 18*, 14–17.

Davidson, H., & Birmingham, C. L. (2001). Letter writing as a therapeutic tool. *Eating and Weight Disorders, 6*, 40-44.

Davin, S. (2003). Healthy viewing: The reception of medical narratives. *Health and media: An overview* [Special issue]. *Sociology of Health & Illness, 25*, 662-679.

Davis, G. A., O'Neill-Pirozzi, T. M., & Coon, M. (1997). Referential cohesion and logical coherence of narration after right hemisphere stroke. *Brain and Language, 56*, 183-210.

Delis, D. C., Wapner, W., Gardner, H., & Moses, J. A., Jr. (1983). The contribution of the right hemisphere to the organization of paragraphs. *Cortex, 19*, 43-50.

Dennis, M. (2001). Inferential language in high-function children with autism. *Journal of Autism and Developmental Disorders, 31*, 47-54.

de Roo, E., Kolk, H., & Hofstede, B. (2002). The ellipsis hypothesis: Syntactically reduced speech of Broca's aphasics and control speakers. *Cortex, 38*, 846-848.

Diamond, S. (2005). Development of expertise in self-management of chronic illness: Narratives of older adults living with atopic dermatitis, and allergies since childhood. *Dissertation Abstracts International, 66*(1-B), 547.

Dijkstra, K., Bourgeois, M., Burgio, L, & Allen, R. (2002). Effects of a communication intervention on the discourse of nursing home residents with dementia and their nursing assistants. *Journal of Medical Speech-Language Pathology, 10*, 143-157.

DiLollo, A., Manning, W., & Neimeyer, R. (2003). Cognitive anxiety as a function of speaker role for fluent speakers and persons who stutter. *Journal of Fluency Disorders, 28*, 167-186.

DiLollo, A., Neimeyer, R., & Manning, W. (2002). A personal construct psychology view of relapse: Indications for a narrative therapy component to stuttering treatment. *Journal of Fluency Disorders, 27*, 19-42.

Dornan, T., Scherpbier, A., King, N., & Boshuizen, H. (2005). Clinical teachers and problem-based learning: A phenomenological study. *Medical Education, 39*, 163-170.

Drew, P. C., & Collins, S. (2001). Conversation analysis: A method for research into interactions between patients and health-care professionals. *Health Expectations: An International Journal of Public Participation in Health Care and Health Policy, 4*, 58-70.

Drew, S. (2003). Self-reconstruction and biographical revisioning: Survival following cancer in childhood or adolescence. *Health: An Interdisciplinary Journal for the Social Study of Health, Illness and Medicine, 7*, 181-199.

Eakin, P. J. (1999). *How our lives become stories: Making selves.* Ithaca, NY: Cornell University Press.

Eggly, S. (2002). Physician-patient co-construction of illness narratives in the medical interview. *Health Communication, 14,* 339–360.

Ehrlich, J. S., Obler, L. K., & Clark, L. (1997). Ideational and semantic contributions to narrative production in adults with dementia of the Alzheimer's type. *Journal of Communication Disorders, 30,* 79–99.

Ellis, C. (1991). Sociological introspection and emotional experience. *Symbolic Interaction, 14,* 23–50.

Ellis, C. (1997). Evocative autoethnography: Writing emotionally about our lives. In W. G. Tierney & Y. S. Lincoln (Eds.), *Representation and the text.* New York: State University of New York Press.

Ellis, C. (2004). *The ethnographic I: A methodological novel about autoethnography.* Walnut Creek, CA: AltaMira Press.

Elman, R. J., Bernstein-Ellis, E., Babbitt, E., Boyle, M., Cherney, L., Fink, R., et al. (2004, November). *A life participation approach to reading: Aphasia book clubs.* Paper presented at the American Speech-Language-Hearing Association Convention, Philadelphia.

Elman, R. J., Bernstein-Ellis, E., Watt, S., Sobel, P., Giuffrida, E., Fink, R., et al. (2005, November). *Reading for pleasure: Aphasia Book Clubs and quality of life.* Paper presented to the American Speech-Language-Hearing Association Convention, San Diego, CA.

Ericsson, K. A., Krampe, R. T., & Tesch-Romer, C. (1993). The role of deliberate practice in the acquisition of expert performance. *Psychological Review, 100,* 363–406.

Faircloth, C. A., Boylstein, C., Young, M. E., & Gubrium, J. (2004). Sudden illness and narrative flow in narratives of stroke recovery. *Sociology of Health and Illness, 26,* 242–261.

Farrington-Darby, T., & Wilson, J. R. (2006). The nature of expertise: A review. *Applied Ergonomics, 37,* 17–32.

Feldman, M. S., Skoldberg, K., Brown, R. N., & Horner, D. (2004). Making sense of stories: A rhetorical approach to narrative analysis. *Journal of Public Administration Research and Theory, 14,* 147–170.

Fernald, L. D. (1987). Of windmills and rope dancing: The instructional value of narrative structures. *Teaching of Psychology, 14*(4), 214–216.

Fernald, L. D. (1994). Tales in a textbook: Learning in the traditional and narrative modes. *Teaching of Psychology, 16*(3), 121–124.

Fick, N. (2006). *One Bullet Away: The Making of Marine Officer.* Boston: Mariner Books.

Floyd, M., Scogin, F., McKendree-Smith, N. L., Floyd, D. L., & Rokke, P. D. (2004). Cognitive therapy for depression: A comparison of individual psychotherapy and bibliotherapy for depressed older adults. *Behavior Modification, 28,* 297–318.

Ford, L. A., & Christman, B. C. (2005). "Every breast cancer is different": Illness narratives and the management of identity in breast cancer. In

E. B. Ray (Ed.), *Health communication in practice: A case study approach*. Mahwah, NJ: Lawrence Erlbaum Associates.

Fox, L. E., Poulson, S. B., & Bowden, K. E. (2004). Critical elements and outcomes of a residential family-based intervention for aphasia caregivers. *Aphasiology, 18*, 1177–1199.

Fraas, M., & Calvert, M. (2006, November. *Oral histories: Bridging misconceptions and reality in brain injury rehabilitation.* Paper presented at the convention of the American Speech-Language-Hearing Association, Miami, FL.

Fraas, M., & Calvert, M. (2006). Stories from a "silent epidemic": Oral history project counters myths about traumatic brain injury. *ASHA Leader, 11*, 10–11, 30.

Frank, A. W. (1991). *At the will of the body: Reflections on illness.* Boston: Houghton Mifflin.

Frank, A. W. (1995). *The wounded storyteller: Body, illness and ethics.* Chicago: University of Chicago Press.

Frank, A. W. (2004). After methods, the story: From incongruity to truth in qualitative research. *Qualitative Health Research, 14*, 430–440.

Frank, E., Breyan, J., & Elon, L. (2000). Physician disclosure of healthy personal behaviors improves credibility and ability to motivate. *Archives of Family Medicine, 9*, 287–290.

Frattali, C., Bayles, K., Beeson, P., Kennedy, M. R. T., Wambaugh, J., & Yorkston, K. (2003). Development of evidence-based practice guidelines: Committee update. *Journal of Medical Speech-Language Pathology, 11*, ix–xviii.

Freeman, M. (2001). From substance to story: Narrative, identity, and the reconstruction of the self. In J. Brockmeier & D. Carbaugh (Eds.) *Narrative and identity: Studies in autobiography, self and culture.* Philadelphia: John Benjamins.

Frieswijk, N., Steverink, N., Buunk, B. P., & Slaets, J. P. J. (2005). The effectiveness of a bibliotherapy in increasing the self-management ability of slightly to moderately frail older people. *Patient Education and Counseling, 61*, 219–227.

Frisini, P. G., Borod, J. C., & Lepore, S. J. (2004). A meta-analysis of the effects of written emotional disclosure on the health outcomes of clinical populations. *The Journal of Nervous and Mental Disease, 192*, 629–634.

Fujiki, M., & Brinton, B. (2005). Foreword: Part 2: Lessons from longitudinal case studies. *Language disorders and learning disabilities: A look across 25 years* [Special issue]. *Topics in Language Disorders, 25*, 337.

Fujiki, M., Brinton, B., & Todd, C. M. (1996). The social skills of children with specific language impairment. *Language, Speech, and Hearing Services in Schools, 27*, 195–202.

Gafaranga, J., & Britten, N. (2003). "Fire away": The opening sequence in general practice consultations. *Family Practice, 20*, 242–247.

Gainotti, G., Caltagironi, C., & Miceli, G. (1983). Selective impairment of semantic-lexical discrimination in right-brain-damaged patients. In E. Perecman (Ed.), *Cognitive processing in the right hemisphere.* New York: Academic Press.

Gallagher, T. J., Hartung, P. J., Herzina, H., Gregory, S. W., & Merolla, D. (2005). Further analysis of a doctor-patient nonverbal communication scale. *Patient Education and Counseling, 57*, 262–271.

Gallant, M. D., & Lafreniere, K. D. (2003). Effects of an emotional disclosure writing task on the physical and psychological functioning of children of alcoholics. *Alcoholism Treatment Quarterly, 21*, 55–66.

Gaver, A., Borkan, J. M., & Weingarten, M. A. (2005). Illness in context and families as teachers: A year-long project for medical students. *Academic Medicine, 80*, 448–451.

Geertz, C. (1988). *Works and lives: The anthropologist as author.* Stanford, CA: Stanford University Press.

Gergen, K. J., & Gergen, M. M. (1986). Narrative form and the construction of psychological science. In T. Sarbin (Ed.), *Narrative psychology: The storied nature of human conduct.* Westport, CT: Praeger.

Golper, L. (2001). ANCDS Practice Guidelines Coordinating Committee report: Proceedings of the Academy of Neurologic Communication Disorders and Sciences. *Journal of Medical Speech-Language Pathology, 9*, ix–x.

Goodman, H. (2001). In-depth interviews. In B. A. Thyer (Ed.), *The handbook of social work research methods.* Thousand Oaks, CA: Sage.

Gorelick, K. (2005). Poetry therapy. In C. A. Malchiodi (Ed.), *Expressive therapies.* New York: Guilford Press.

Gornick, V. (2001). *The situation and the story: The art of personal narrative.* New York: Farrar, Strauss & Giroux.

Graybeal, A. (2004). Expressive 2,writing as a therapeutic intervention for adult children of divorce [electronic resource]. Doctoral dissertation, The University of Texas at Austin. Available electronically from http://hdl.handle.net/2152/112

Greenhalgh, T., & Collard, A. (2003). *Narrative based health care: Sharing stories. A multiprofessional workbook.* London: BMJ.

Greenhalgh, T., & Hurwitz, B. (Eds.). (1998). *Narrative-based medicine: Dialogue and discourse in clinical practice.* London: BMJ.

Greenhalgh, T., Robert, G., Macfarlane, F., Bate, P., Kyriakidou, O., & Peacock, R. (2005). Storylines of research in diffusion of innovation: A meta-narrative approach to systematic review. *Social Science & Medicine, 61*, 417–430.

Grinyer, A. (2004). The narrative correspondence method: What a follow-up study can tell us about the longer term effect on participants in emotionally demanding research. *Building theory* [Special issue]. *Qualitative Health Research, 14,* 1326–1341.

Guendouzi, J., & Muller, N. (2006). *Approaches to discourse in dementia.* Mahwah, NJ: Lawrence Erlbaum.

Guilford, A. M., Graham, S. V., & Scheuerle, J. (Eds.). (2007). *The speech-language pathologist: From novice to expert.* New York: Pearson Merrill/Prentice-Hall.

Hall, W. A. (1961). Return from silence: A personal experience. *Journal of Speech and Hearing Disorders, 26,* 174–176.

Halper, A. S., Cherney, L. R. & Miller, T. K. (1991). *Clinical Management of Communication Problems in Adults with Traumatic Brain Injury.* New York: Aspen.

Hardy, B. (1986). Towards a poetics of fiction: An approach through narrative. *Novel, 2,* 5–14.

Harper, D. (2004). Introducing social constructionist and critical psychology into clinical psychology training. In D. A. Pare & G. Larner (Eds.), *Collaborative practice in psychology and therapy.* New York: Haworth Press.

Harris, A. H. (2004). Effects of expressive writing on lung function in adult asthmatics. *Dissertation Abstracts International, 64*(11-B), 2310.

Hatch, J. A. (2002). *Doing qualitative research in education settings.* Albany, NY: State University of New York Press.

Hatem, D., & Rider, E. A. (2004). Sharing stories: Narrative medicine in an evidence-based world. *Patient Education & Counseling, 54,* 251–253.

Hemphill, L., Feldman, H. M., & Camp, L. (1994). Developmental changes in narrative and non-narrative discourse in children with and without brain injury. *Journal of Communication Disorders, 27,* 107–133.

Heritage, J., & Maynard, D. W. (2005). *Communication in medical care: Interactions between primary care physicians and patients.* Cambridge, UK: Cambridge University Press.

Hermans, H. J. M. (1996). Self-narrative in the life course: A contextualized approach. In M. Bamberg (Ed.), *Narrative development: Six approaches.* Mahwah, NJ: Lawrence Erlbaum Associates.

Hersch, D. (2001). Experiences of ending aphasia therapy. *International Journal of Language & Communication Disorders, 36,* 80–85.

Hersch, D. (2003). "Weaning" clients from aphasia therapy: Speech pathologists' strategies for discharge. *Aphasiology, 17,* 1007–1029.

Hill, J. H. (2005). Finding culture in narrative. In N. Quinn (Ed.), *Finding culture in talk.* New York: Palgrave Macmillan.

Hinckley, J. J. (2000). *What is it like to have a communication impairment? Simulation for family, friends and caregivers.* Stow, OH: Interactive Therapeutics.

Hinckley, J. J. (2006). Finding messages in bottles: Living successfully with stroke and aphasia. *Topics in Stroke Rehabilitation, 13,* 25–36.

Hinckley, J. J. (2007). Problem-solving and treatment integrity. In A. M. Guilford, S. Graham, & J. Scheuerle (Eds.), *The speech-language pathologist: From novice to expert*. New York: Pearson Merrill/Prentice-Hall.

Hinckley, J. J., Craig, H. K., & Anderson, L. A. (1989). Communication characteristics of physician-patient information exchanges. In Giles, H. & Robinson, W. P. (Eds.), *Handbook of language and social psychology* (pp. 519–536). London: Wiley.

Honda, R., Mitachi, M., & Watamori, T. S. (1999). Production of discourse of high-functioning individuals with aphasia—with reference to performance on the Japanese CADL. *Aphasiology, 13*, 475–493.

Hopper, T., Holland, A., & Rewega, M. (2002). Conversational coaching: Treatment outcomes and future directions. *Aphasiology, 16*, 745–761.

Horton, S., & Byng, S. (2000). Examining interaction in aphasia therapy. *International Journal of Language & Communication Disorders, 35*, 355–375.

Hoshmand, L. T. (2000). Narrative psychology. In A. E. Kazdin (Ed.), *Encyclopedia of psychology* (Vol. 5, pp. 382–387). Washington, DC: American Psychological Association.

Hough, M. S., & Pierce, R. S. (1993). Contextual and thematic influences on narrative comprehension of left and right hemisphere brain-damaged adults. In H. Brownell & Y. Joanette (Eds.), *Narrative discourse in neurologically impaired and normal aging adults* (pp. 213–238). San Diego, CA: Singular.

Hughes, J. C., Louw, S. T., & Sabat, S. R. (2006). *Dementia: Mind, meaning, and the person*. New York: Oxford University Press.

Hunter, K. M. (1986). "There was this one guy . . . ": The uses of anecdotes in medicine. *Perspectives in Biology and Medicine, 29*, 619–630.

Iedema, R., Flabouris, A., Grant, S., & Jorm, C. (2006). Narrativizing errors of care: Critical incident reporting in clinical practice. *Social Science & Medicine, 62*, 134–144.

Joanette, Y., Goulet, P., Ska, B., & Nespoulous, J. (1986). Informative content of narrative discourse in right-brain-damaged right-handers. *Brain and Language, 29*, 81–105.

Joanette, Y., Lecours, A. R., Lepage, Y., & Lamoureux, M. (1983). Language in right-handers with right-hemisphere lesions: A preliminary study including anatomical, genetic, and social factors. *Brain and Language, 20*, 217–248.

Johnson, C. J. (2006). Getting started in evidence-based practice in childhood language disorders. *American Journal of Speech-Language Pathology, 15*, 20–35.

Johnston, J., Miller, J., & Tallal, P. (2001). Use of cognitive state predicates by language-impaired children. *International Journal of Language & Communication Disorders, 36*, 349–370.

Jones, A. C. (2004). Transforming the story: Narrative applications to a stepmother support group. *Families in Society, 85*, 129-138.

Josselson, R. (2004). On becoming the narrator of one's own life. In D. P. McAdams (Ed.), *Healing plots: The narrative basis of psychotherapy* (pp. 111-129). Washington, DC: American Psychological Association.

Juncos-Rabadan, O., Pereiro, A. X., & Rodriguez, M. S. (2005). Narrative speech in aging: Quantity, information content, and cohesion. *Brain and Language, 95*, 423-434.

Kadaravek, J. N., Gillam, R. B., Ukrainetz, T. A., Justice, L. M., & Eisenberg, S. N. (2004). School-age children's self-assessment of oral narrative production. *Communication Disorders Quarterly, 26*, 37-48.

Kathard, H. (2001). Sharing stories: Life history narratives in stuttering research. *International Journal of Language & Communication Disorders, 36*(Suppl.), 52-57.

Kern, D. E., Branch, W. T., Jackson, J. L., Brady, D. W., Feldman, M. D., Levinson, W., et al. (2005). Teaching the psychosocial aspects of care in the clinical setting: Practical recommendations. *Academic Medicine, 80*, 8-20.

Kim, E. S., Cleary, S. J., Hopper, T., Bayles, K. A., Mahendra, N., Azuma, T., et al. (2006). Evidence-based practice recommendations for working with individuals with dementia: Group reminiscence therapy. *Journal of Medical Speech-Language Pathology, 14*, 23-35.

King, J. T., Yonas, H., Horowitz, M. B., Kassam, A. B., & Roberts, M. S. (2005). A failure to communicate: Patients with cerebral aneurysms and vascular neurosurgeons. *Journal of Neurology, Neurosurgery & Psychiatry, 76*(4), 550-554.

Kovac, S. H., & Range, L. M. (2002). Does writing about suicidal thoughts and feelings reduce them? *Suicide and Life-Threatening Behavior, 32*, 428-440.

Landis, B. F. (2004). A simple pen to paper: What's the big deal? *Home Health Care Management and Practice, 16*, 512-517.

László, J. (2004). Narrative psychology's contribution to the second cognitive revolution. *Journal of Cultural and Evolutionary Psychology, 2*, 337-354.

Laub, D. (2006). From speechlessness to narrative: The cases of holocaust historians and of psychiatrically hospitalized survivors. *Literature and Medicine, 24*, 253-265.

Law, J., Garrett, Z., & Nye, C. (2004). The efficacy of treatment for chidren with developmental language delay/disorder: A meta-analysis. *Journal of Speech, Language, & Hearing Research, 47*, 924-943.

Leahy, M. (2004). Therapy talk: Analyzing therapeutic discourse. *Language, Speech, and Hearing Services in Schools, 35*, 70-81.

Lee, A. M., & Poole, G. (2005). An application of the transactional model to the analysis of chronic illness narratives. *Qualitative Health Research*, *15*, 346-364.

Lee, C. (2004). Agency and purpose in narrative therapy: Questioning the postmodern rejection of metanarrative. *Journal of Psychology and Theology*, *32*, 221-231.

Lepore, S. J., & Smyth, J. M. (Eds.). (2002). *The writing cure: How expressive writing promotes health and emotional well-being*. Washington, DC: American Psychological Association.

Leys, D., Lejeune, J. P., & Pruvo, J. P. (2005). A failure to communicate: Patients with cerebral aneurysms and vascular neurosurgeons: Comment. *Journal of Neurology, Neurosurgery & Psychiatry*, *76*, 467-468.

Li, E. C., Williams, S. E., & Della Volpe, A. (1995). The effects of topic and listener familiarity on discourse variables in procedural and narrative discourse tasks. *Journal of Communication Disorders*, *28*, 39-55.

Li, H. Z. (2001). Cooperative and intrusive interruptions in inter- and intracultural dyads. *Journal of Language and Social Psychology*, *20*, 259-284.

Liles, B. Z. (1985). Production and comprehension of narrative discourse in normal and language disordered children. *Journal of Communication Disorders*, *18*, 409-427.

Liles, B. Z. (1993). Narrative discourse in children with language disorders and children with normal language: A critical review of the literature. *Journal of Speech and Hearing Research*, *36*, 868-882.

Logan, G. D. (1988). Toward an instance theory of automaticity. *Psychological Review*, *95*, 492-527.

Logan, G. D. (2002). An instance theory of attention and memory. *Psychological Review*, *109*, 376-400.

Lyon, J. G., Cariski, D., Keisler, L., Rosenbek, J., Levine, R., Kumpula, J., et al. (1997). Communication partners: Enhancing participation in life and communication for adults with aphasia in natural settings. *Aphasiology*, *11*, 693-708.

Mann, T. (2001). Effects of future writing and optimism on health behaviors in HIV-infected women. *Annals of Behavioral Medicine*, *23*, 26-33.

Maruna, S. (1997). Going straight: Desistance from crime and life narratives of reform. In A. Lieblich & R. Josselson (Eds.), *The narrative study of lives* (pp. 59-97). Thousand Oaks, CA: Sage.

Mateas, M. & Sengers, P. (2003). Narrative intelligence. In: Mateas, M. & Sengers, P. (Eds.), *Narrative Intelligence*. Amsterdam, Netherlands: John Benjamins.

Maynard, D. W., & Heritage, J. (2005). Conversation analysis, doctor-patient interaction and medical communication. *Medical Education*, *39*, 428-435.

McAdams, D. P. (1984). Love, power, and images of the self. In C. Z. Malatesta & C. E. Izard (Eds.), *Emotion in adult development* (pp. 159-174). Beverly Hills, CA: Sage.

McAdams, D. P. (1993). *The stories we live by: Personal myths and the making of the self.* New York: Guilford Press.

McAdams, D. P. (1996). Personality, modernity, and the storied self: A contemporary framework for studying persons. *Psychological Inquiry, 7,* 295-321.

McAdams, D. P. (1999). Personal narratives and the life story. In L. Pervin & O. John (Eds.), *Handbook of personality: Theory and research* (2nd ed., pp 478-500.). New York: Guilford.

McAdams, D. P. (2003). Identity and the life story. In R. Fivush & C. A. Haden (Eds.), *Autobiographical memory and the construction of a narrative self: Developmental and cultural perspectives* (pp. 187-207). Mahwah, NJ: Lawrence Erlbaum.

McAdams, D. P., de St. Aubin, E., & Logan, R. (1993). Generativity among young, midlife, and older adults. *Psychology and Aging, 8,* 221-230.

McAdams, D. P., Diamond, A., de St. Aubin, E., & Manfield, E. (1997). Stories of commitment: The psychosocial construction of generative lives. *Journal of Personality and Social Psychology, 72,* 678-694.

McAdams, D. P., Josselson, R., & Lieblich, A. (Eds.). (2001). *Turns in the road: Narrative studies of lives in transition* (pp.). Washington, DC: American Psychological Association.

McArdle, S., & Byrt, R. (2001). Fiction, poetry and mental health: Expressive and therapeutic uses of literature. *Journal of Psychiatric and Mental Health Nursing, 8,* 517-524.

McBride, H. E. A., & Siegel, L. S. (1997). Learning disabilities and adolescent suicide. *Journal of Learning Disabilities, 39,* 652-659.

McCabe, A., & Peterson, C. (Eds.). (1991). *Developing narrative structure* (pp.). Hillsdale, NJ: Lawrence Erlbaum.

McCarthy, J., Donofrio, L., Dempsey, L., Birr, K., & Pratt, S. (2006, November). *Influence of personal narratives on businesspeople's attitudes toward AAC users.* Paper presented at the convention of the American Speech-Language-Hearing Association, Miami, FL.

McColl, M. (2003). Illness stories: Themes emerging through narrative. *Social Work in Health Care, 37*(1), 19-39.

McCrum, R. (1999). *My year off: Recovering life after a stroke.* New York: Broadway Books.

McDonald, S. (1993). Pragmatic language abilities after closed head injury: Ability to meet the informational needs of the listener. *Brain and Language, 44,* 24-86.

McDonald, S. (2000). Exploring the cognitive basis of right-hemisphere pragmatic language disorder. *Brain and Language, 75,* 82-107.

McEvoy, M. A., Shores, R. E., Wehby, J. H., Johnson, S. M., & Fox, J. J. (1990). Special education teachers' implementation of procedures to promote social interaction among children in integrated settings. *Education and Training in Mental Retardation, 25,* 267–276.

McGannon, K. R. (2002). Toward an alternative theory of self and identity for understanding and investigating adherence to exercise and physical activity. *Dissertation Abstracts International, 63*(5-A), 1766.

McQuiston, C., Parrado, E. A., Colmos-Muniz, J. C. & Bustillo Martinez, A. M. (2005). Community-based participatory research and ethnography: The perfect union. In B. A. Israel, E. Eng, A. J. U. Schulz, & E. A. Parker (Eds.), *Methods in Community-Based Participatory Research for Health.* San Francisco: Jossey-Bass.

Meichenbaum, D. (2006). Trauma and suicide: A constructive narrative perspective. In T. E. Ellis (Ed.), *Cognition and suicide: Theory, research, and therapy* (pp. 356–377). Washington, DC: American Psychological Association.

Milan, F. B., Parish, S. J., & Reichgott, M. J. (2006). A model for educational feedback based on clinical communication skills strategies: Beyond the "feedback sandwich." *Teaching and Learning in Medicine, 18,* 42–47.

Miller, W. L., & Crabtree, B. F. (2003). Clinical research. In N. K. Denzin & Y. S. Lincoln (Eds.), *Strategies of qualitative inquiry* (2nd ed., pp. 607–621). Thousand Oaks, CA: Sage.

Mishler, E. (1986). *Research interviewing: Context and narrative.* Cambridge, MA: Harvard University Press.

Mishler, E. G. (2004). Historians of the self: Restorying lives, revising identities. *Research in Human Development, 1,* 101–121.

Mittelman, M.S., Ferris, S. H., Shulman, E., Steinberg, G., Mackell, J., & Ambinder, A., (1994). Efficacy of multicomponenet individualized treatment to improve the well-being of Alzheimer's caregivers. In Light, E., Niederehe, G., & Lebowitz, B. D. (Eds.), *Stress effects on family caregivers of Alzheimer's patients: Research and interventions (*pp. 95–109*).* New York: Springer.

Montbriand, M. J. (2004). Seniors' life histories and perceptions of illness. *Western Journal of Nursing Research, 26,* 242–260.

Morgan-Witte, J. (2005). Narrative knowledge development among caregivers: Stories from the nurses' station. In L. M. Harter, P. M. Japp,.& C. S. Beck (Eds.), *Narratives, health, and healing: Communication theory, research, and practice* (pp. 217–236). Mahwah, NJ: Lawrence Erlbaum Associates.

Moss, B., Parr, S., Byng, S., & Petheram, B. (2004). "Pick me up and not a down down, up up": How are the identities of people with aphasia represented in aphasia, stroke and disability websites? *Disability & Society, 19,* 753–768.

Moss, B., & Roberts, C. (2005). Explanations, explanations, explanations: How do patients with limited English construct narrative accounts in multi-lingual, multi-ethnic settings, and how can GPs interpret them? *Family Practice, 22*, 412-418.

Moya, K. L., Benowitz, L. I., Levine, D. N., & Finklestein, S. (1986). Covariant defects in visuospatial abilities and recall of verbal narrative after right hemisphere stroke. *Cortex, 22*, 381-397.

Murray, L .L. (2000). Spoken language production in Huntington's and Parkinson's diseases. *Journal of Speech, Language, and Hearing Research, 43*, 1350-1366.

Murray, M. (2003). Narrative psychology. In J. A. Smith (Ed.), *Qualitative psychology: A practical guide to research methods* (pp. 256-277). Thousand Oaks, CA: Sage.

Murray, M. (2003). Narrative psychology and narrative analysis. In P. M. Camic, J. E. Rhodes, & L. Yardley (Eds.), *Qualitative research in psychology: Expanding perspectives in methodology and design* (pp. 95-112). Washington, DC: American Psychological Association.

Myers, G. E. (2002). Can illness narratives contribute to the delay of hospice admission? *American Journal of Hospice & Palliative Care, 19*, 325-330.

Myers, P. S. (1993). Narrative expressive deficits associated with right-hemisphere damage. In H. Brownell & Y. Joanette (Eds.), *Narrative discourse in neurologically impaired and normal aging adults* (pp. 153-169). San Diego, CA: Singular.

Myers, P. S. (1997). Right hemisphere syndrome. In L. LaPointe (Ed.), *Aphasia and related neurogenic language disorders* (2nd ed., pp. 232-255). New York: Thieme.

Naigles, L. R. (2001). Manipulating the input: Studies in mental verb acquisition. In B. Landau, J. Sabini, J. Jonides, & E. L. Newport (Eds.), *Perception, cognition, and language: Essays in honor of Henry and Lila Gleitman* (pp. 123-144). Cambridge, MA: MIT Press.

Nast, P. A., Avidan, M., Harris, C. B., Krauss, M. J., Jacobson, E., Petlin, A., et al. (2005). Reporting and classification of patient safety events in a cardiothoracic intensive care unit and cardiothoracic postoperative care unit. *The Journal of Thoracic and Cardiovascular Surgery, 130*, 1137.

Neiser, U. (Ed.). (1993). *The perceived self.* New York: Cambridge University Press.

Neiser, U., & Fivush, R. (1996). *The remembered self: Accuracy and construction in the life narrative.* New York: Cambridge University Press.

Neiser, U., & Jopling, D. (1997). *The conceptual self in context: Culture, experience, self-understanding.* New York: Cambridge University Press.

Nelson, K. (1993). The psychological and social origins of autobiographical memory. *Psychological Science, 4*, 7-14.

Nettlebeck, T., & Kirby, N. H. (1976). A comparison of part and whole training methods with mildly mentally retarded workers. *Journal of Occupational Psychology, 49,* 115-120.

Nicholas, L. E., & Brookshire, R. H. (1993). A system for quantifying the informativeness and efficiency of the connected speech in adults with aphasia. *Journal of Speech and Hearing Research, 36,* 338-350.

Noell, G. H., Gresham, F. M., & Gansle, K. A. (2002). Does treatment integrity matter? A preliminary investigation of instructional implementation and mathematics performance. *Journal of Behavioral Education, 11,* 51-67.

Norbury, C. F., & Bishop, D. V. M. (2003). Narrative skills of children with communication impairments. *International Journal of Language & Communication Disorders, 38,* 287-313.

North, A. J., Ulatowska, H. K., Macaluso-Haynes, S., & Bell, H. (1986). Discourse impairments in older adults. *International Journal of Aging and Human Development, 23,* 267-286.

Norton, C. S. (1989). *Life metaphors: Stories of ordinary survival.* Carbondale: Southern Illinois Press.

Nuessel, F., & Van Stewart, A. (1999). Literary exemplars of illness: A strategy for personalizing geriatric case histories in clinical settings. *Physical & Occupational Therapy in Geriatrics, 16,* 33-53.

Ochberg, R. L. (1996). Interpreting life stories. In R. Josselson (Ed.), *Narrative study of lives* (Vol. 4, pp.). Thousand Oaks, CA: Sage.

Okely, J. (1996). *Own or other culture.* New York: Routledge.

Olney, J. (1998). *Memory and narrative: The weave of life writing.* Chicago: University of Chicago Press.

Olsen, R. A. (2005). Free will and therapeutic change. *Pastoral Psychology, 53,* 267-279.

O'Sullivan, M., & Doutis, P. (1994). Research on expertise: Guideposts for expertise and teacher education in physical education. *QUEST, 46,* 176-185.

Pamphilon, B. (2005). How aged women remember their life-long/life-wide learning: Making the best of life. *Educational Gerontology, 31,* 283-299.

Pasupathi, M. (2006). Silk from sows' ears: Collaborative construction of everyday selves in everyday stories. In D. P. McAdams, R. Josselson, & A. Lieblich (Eds.), *Identity and story: Creating self in narrative* (pp. 129-150). Washington, DC: American Psychological Association.

Pennebaker, J. W. (1997). *Opening up: The healing power of expressing emotions.* New York: Guilford Press.

Pennebaker, J. W. (Ed.). (2002). *Emotion, disclosure, and health.* New York: American Psychological Association.

Pennebaker, J. W. (2004). *Writing to heal: A guided journal for recovering from trauma and emotional upheaval.* Oakland, CA: New Harbinger Press.

Pennebaker, J. W., & Graybeal, A. (2001). Patterns of natural language use: Disclosure, personality, and social integration. *Current Directions in Psychological Science, 10,* 90-93.

Pennebaker, J. W., Mayne, T. J., & Francis, M. E. (1997). Linguistic predictors of adaptive bereavement. *Journal of Personality and Social Psychology, 72,* 863-871.

Pennebaker, J. W., & Seagal, J. D. (1999). Forming a story: The health benefits of narrative. *Journal of Clinical Psychology, 55,* 1243-1254.

Perez, P. (2001). *Brain attack: Danger, chaos, opportunity, empowerment.* Johnson, VT: Cutting Edge Press.

Petersen, S., Bull, C., Probst, O., Dettinger, S., & Detwiler, L. (2005). Narrative therapy to prevent illness-related stress disorder. *Journal of Counseling and Development, 83,* 41-47.

Peterson, C. C., & Slaughter, V. P. (2006). Telling the story of theory of mind: Deaf and hearing children's narratives and mental state understanding. *British Journal of Developmental Psychology, 24,* 151-179.

Petrie, K. J., Fontanilla, I., Thomas, M. G., Booth, R. J., & Pennebaker, J. W. (2004). Effect of written emotional expression on immune function in patients with human immunodeficiency virus infection: A randomized trial. *Psychosomatic Medicine, 66,* 272-275.

Phinney, A. (2002). Fluctuating awareness and the breakdown of the illness narrative in dementia. *Dementia: The International Journal of Social Research and Practice, 1,* 329-344.

Pillemer, D. B. (1998). *Momentous events, vivid memories.* Cambridge, MA: Harvard University Press.

Polkinghorne, D. (1995). Narrative configuration in qualitative analysis. In J. A. Hatch & R. Wisniewski (Eds.), *Life history and narrative.* London: Falmer Press.

Portnuff, C. (2006). A partnership for communication: A personal journey through amyotrophic lateral sclerosis. *ASHA Leader, 11*(6), 32-33.

Pound, C., Parr, S., & Duchan, J. (2001). Using partners' autobiographical reports to develop, deliver, and evaluate services in aphasia. *Aphasiology, 15,* 477-493.

Pound, C., Parr, S., Lindsay, J., & Woolf, C. (2000). *Beyond aphasia: Therapies for living with communication disability.* Brackley, UK: Speechmark.

Preece, A. (1987). The range of narrative forms conversationally produced by young children. *Journal of Child Language, 14,* 353-373.

Prince, S., Haynes, W. O., & Haak, N. J. (2002). Occurrence of contingent queries and discourse errors in referential communication and conversational tasks: A study of college students with closed head injury. *Journal of Medical Speech-Language Pathology, 10*, 19-39.

Prochaska, J. O. (1994). Strong and weak principles for progressing from precontemplation to action on the basis of twelve problem behaviors. *Health Psychology, 13*, 47-51.

Prochaska, J., & DiClemente, C. (1984). *The transtheoretical approach: Crossing traditional boundaries of therapy.* Homewood, IL: Dow Jones-Irwin.

Prochaska, J. O., & Velicer, W. F. (1997). The transtheoretical model of health behavior change. *American Journal of Health Promotion, 12*, 38-48.

Pullman, D., Bethune, C., & Duke, P. (2005). Narrative means to humanistic ends. *Teaching and Learning in Medicine, 17*, 279-284.

Quinn, N. (2005). *Finding culture in talk.* New York: Palgrave Macmillan.

Redman, R. W. (2005). The power of narrative. *Research and Theory for Nursing Practice: An International Journal, 19*, 5-7.

Reed-Danahay, D. E. (Ed.). (1997). *Auto/ethnography: Rewriting the self and the social.* Oxford, UK: Berg.

Rich, M., & Patashnick, J. (2002). Narrative research with audiovisual data: Video intervention/prevention assessment (VIA) and NVivo. *Qualitative research and computing: Methodological issues and practices in using QSR NVivo and NUDIST* [Special issue]. *International Journal of Social Research Methodology: Theory & Practice, 5*, 245-261.

Rich, P., & Copans, S. A. (1998). *The healing journey: Your journal of self-discovery.* Hoboken, NJ: John Wiley & Sons.

Ricoeur, P. (1983). *Time and narrative.* Chicago: University of Chicago Press.

Ricoeur, P. (1991). The human experience of time and narrative. In M. Waldes (Ed.), *A Ricoeur reader: Reflection and imagination.* New York: Harvester Wheatsheaf.

Riediger, M., Freund, A. M., & Baltes, P. B. (2005). Managing life through personal goals: Intergoal facilitation and intensity of goal pursuit in younger and older adulthood. *Journals of Gerontology, Series B: Psychological Sciences and Social Sciences, 60B*, P84-P91.

Riessman, C. K. (1993). *Narrative analysis.* London: Sage.

Riessman, C. K., & Quinney, L. (2005). Narrative in social work: A critical review. *Qualitative Social Work: Research and Practice, 4*, 391-412.

Riley, T., & Hawe, P. (2005). Researching practice: The methodological case for narrative inquiry. *Health Education Research, 20*, 226-236.

Ripich, D. N. (1989). Children's perceptions of roles in intervention. *Journal of Childhood Communication Disorders, 12*, 127-136.

Robey, R., & Dalebout, S. (1998). A tutorial on conducting meta-analyses of clinical outcome research. *Journal of Speech, Language & Hearing Research, 41*, 1227-1241.

Roper, J. M., & Shapira, J. (2000). *Ethnography in nursing research.* Thousand Oaks, CA: Sage.

Rosenberg, S. D., Rosenberg, H. J., & Farrell, M. P. (1999). The midlife crisis revisited. In S. L. Willis & J. D. Reid (Eds.), *Life in the middle: Psychological and social development in middle age* (pp. 47-73). San Diego, CA: Academic Press.

Rosenthal, G. (2003). The healing effects of storytelling: On the conditions of curative storytelling in the context of research and counseling. *Qualitative Inquiry, 9,* 915-933.

Rosenwald, G., & Ochberg, R. (Eds.). (1992). *Storied lives: The cultural politics of self-understanding.* New Haven, CT: Yale University Press.

Rosenwald, G. C. (1996). Making whole: Method and ethics in mainstream and narrative psychology. In R. Josselson (Ed.), *Ethics and process in the narrative study of lives* (pp. 245-273). Thousand Oaks, CA: Sage.

Ross, K. B., & Wertz, R. T. (1999). Comparison of impairment and disability measures for assessing severity of, and improvement in, aphasia. *Aphasiology, 13,* 113-124.

Rowland-Morin, P. A., & Carroll, J. (1990). Verbal communication skills and patient satisfaction: A study of doctor-patient interviews. *Evaluation and the Health Professions, 13,* 168-185.

Rubin, S., Bicklen, D., Kasa-Hendrickson, C., Bluth, P., Cardinal, D. N., & Broderick, A. (2001). Independence, participation, and the meaning of intellectual ability. *Disability & Society, 16,* 415-429.

Sackett, D. L., Rosenberg, W. M. C., Gray, J. A. M., Haynes, R. B., & Richardson, W. S. (1996). Evidence-based medicine: What it is and what it isn't: It's about integrating individual clinical expertise with the best external evidence. *British Medical Journal, 312,* 711-712.

Sackett, D. L., Straus, S. E., Richardson, W. S., Rosenberg, W., & Haynes, R. B. (2000). *Evidence-based medicine: How to practice and teach EBM* (2nd ed.). Edinburgh, UK: Churchill Livingstone.

Saffran, E. M., Berndt, R. S., & Schwartz, M. F. (1989). The quantitative analysis of agrammatic production: Procedure and data. *Brain and Language, 37,* 440-479.

Sage, R. (2005). Communicating with students who have learning and behaviour difficulties: A continuing professional development programme. *Emotional & Behavioural Difficulties, 10,* 281-297.

Sarbin, T. R. (1986). The narrative as a root metaphor for psychotherapy. In T. R. Sarbin (Ed.), *Narrative psychology: The storied nature of human conduct.* Westport, CT: Praeger.

Schafer, R. (2004). Narrating, attending, empathizing. *Literature and Medicine, 23,* 241-251.

Schank, R. C. (1991). *Tell me a story: A new look at real and artificial intelligence.* New York: Simon & Schuster.

Schank, R. C., & Abelson, R. (1977). *Scripts, plans, goals, and understanding.* Hillsdale, NJ: Erlbaum Associates.

Schank, R. C., & Abelson, R. P. (1995). Knowledge and memory: The real story. In R. S. Wyer, Jr. (Ed.), *Knowledge and memory: The real story* (pp. 1–85). Hillsdale, NJ: Lawrence Erlbaum Associates.

Schiffrin, D. (1996). Narrative as self-portrait: Sociolinguistic constructions of identity. *Language in Society, 25,* 167–203.

Schnell, L. J. (2004). Learning how to tell. *Literature and Medicine, 23,* 265–279.

Schulz, R., Williamson, G. M., & Morycz, R. (1993). Changes in depression among men and women caring for an Alzheimer's patient. In S. H. Zarit, L. I. Pearlin, & K. W. Schaie (Eds.), *Caregiving systems: Formal and informal helpers* (pp. 152–171). Hillsdale, NJ: Lawrence Erlbaum.

Schwartz, L., & Drotar, D. (2004). Linguistic analysis of written narratives of caregivers of children and adolescents with chronic illness: Cognitive and emotional processes and physical and psychological health outcomes. *Journal of Clinical Psychology in Medical Settings, 11,* 291–301.

Seidman, I. (2006). *Interviewing as qualitative research: A guide for researchers in education and the social sciences* (3rd ed.). New York: Teachers College Press.

Sells, D., Topor, A., & Davidson, L. (2004). Generating coherence out of chaos: Examples of the utility of empathic bridges in phenomenological research. *Phenomenology and Contemporary Clinical Practice* [Special issue]. *Journal of Phenomenological Psychology, 35*(2), 253–271.

Semple, C. J., Dunwoody, L., Sullivan, K., & Kernohan, W. G. (2006). Patients with head and neck cancer prefer individualized cognitive behavioural therapy. *European Journal of Cancer Care, 15,* 220–227.

Sengers, P. (2000). Narrative intelligence. In K. Dautenhahn (Ed.), *Human cognition and social agent technology* (pp. 1–26). Amsterdam, Netherlands: John Benjamins.

Sengers, P. (2003). Schizophrenia and narrative in artificial agents. In M. Mateas & P. Sengers (Eds.), *Narrative intelligence* (pp. 427–431). Amsterdam, Netherlands: John Benjamins.

Shadden, B. (2005). Aphasia as identity theft: Theory and practice. *Aphasiology, 19,* 211–223.

Shanteau, J. (1992). The psychology of experts: An alternative view. In G. Wright & F. Bolger (Eds.), *Expertise and decision support* (pp. 11–23). New York: Plenum Press.

Sharf, B. F. (2005). How I fired my surgeon and embraced an alternative narrative. In L. M. Harter, P. M. Japp, & C. S. Beck (Eds.), *Narratives, health, and healing: Communication theory, research, and practice* (pp. 325–342). Mahwah, NJ: Lawrence Erlbaum Associates.

Silliman, E. R., Diehl, S. F., Bahr, R. H., Hnath-Chisolm, T., Zenko, C. B., & Friedman, S. A. (2003). A new look at performance on theory-of-mind tasks by adolescents with autism spectrum disorder. *Language, Speech, and Hearing Services in Schools, 34*, 236-282.

Silverberg, L. I. (2003). Bibliotherapy: The therapeutic use of didactic and literary texts in treatment, diagnosis, prevention, and training. *The Journal of the American Osteopathic Association, 103*, 131-135.

Simmons-Mackie, N., & Damico, J. S. (1999). Social role negotiation in aphasia therapy: Competence, incompetence and conflict. In D. Kovarsky, J. F. Duchan, & M. Maxwell (Eds.), *Constructing (in) competence: Disabling evaluations in clinical and social interaction* (pp. 313-341). Mahwah, NJ: Lawrence Erlbaum Associates.

Simmons-Mackie, N., & Schultz, M. (2003). The role of humour in therapy for aphasia. *Aphasiology, 17*, 751-766.

Simpson, G., & Tate, R. (2005). Clinical features of suicide attempts after traumatic brain injury. *Journal of Nervous and Mental Disease, 193*, 680-685.

Singer, J. A., & Moffitt, K. H. (1991-1992). An experimental investigation of specificity and generality in memory narratives. *Imagination, Cognition, and Personality, 11*, 233-257.

Singer, J. A., & Salovey, P. (1993). *The remembered self: Emotion and memory in personality.* New York: The Free Press.

Singer, J. A., & Singer, J. L. (1994). Social-cognitive and narrative perspectives on transference. In J. Masling & R. F. Bornstein (Eds.), *Empirical perspectives on object relations theory* (pp. 157-194). Washington, DC: American Psychological Association.

Skultans, V. A. (1997). A historical disorder: Neurasthenia and the testimony of lives. *Anthropological Medicine, 4*, 7-24.

Skultans, V. (1997). *The testimony of lives: Narrative and memory in post-Soviet Latvia.* London: Routledge.

Skultans, V. (1998). Anthropology and narrative. In T. Greenhalgh & B. Hurwitz (Eds.), *Narrative-based medicine: Dialogue and discourse in clinical practice* (pp. 42-53). London: BMJ.

Snow, P., Douglas, J., & Ponsford, J. (1998). Conversational discourse abilities following severe traumatic brain injury: A follow-up study. *Brain Injury, 12*, 911-935.

Solbakk, J. H. (2004). Therapeutic doubt and moral dialogue. *The Journal of Medicine and Philosophy, 29*, 93-119.

Soto, G., & Harman, E. (2006). Analysis of narratives produced by four children who use augmentative and alternative communication. *Journal of Communication Disorders, 39*, 456-480.

Sparkes, A. C. (2000). Autoethnography and narratives of self: Reflections on criteria in action. *Sociology of Sport Journal, 17*, 21-41.

Spilkin, M. L. (2003). A conversation analysis approach to facilitating communication with memory books. *Advances in Speech-Language Pathology, 5*, 105–118.

Spradley, J. P. (1979). *The ethnographic interview.* New York: Holt, Rinehart and Winston.

Spry, T. (2001). Performing autoethnography: An embodied methodological praxis. *Qualitative Inquiry, 7*, 706–732.

Sridhar, D., & Vaughn, S. (2002). Bibliotherapy: Practices for improving self-concept and reading comprehension. In B. Y. L. Wong & M. Donahue (Eds.), *The social dimensions of learning disabilities: Essays in honor of Tanis Bryan* (pp. 161–185). Mahwah, NJ: Lawrence Erlbaum.

Stein, H. F. (2004). A window to the interior of experience. *Families, Systems & Health, 22*, 178–179.

Stern, L., & Kirmayer, L. J. (2004). Knowledge structures in illness narratives: Development and reliability of a coding scheme. *Transcultural Psychiatry, 41*, 130–142.

Stevenson, R. L. (1988). *The lantern-bearers and other essays.* New York: Farrar Strauss Giroux.

Stiegler, L. N., & Hoffman, P. R. (2001). Discourse-based intervention for word finding in children. *Journal of Communication Disorders, 34*, 277–303.

Stout, C. E., Yorkston, K. M., & Pimentel, J. I. (2000). Discourse production following mild, moderate, and severe traumatic brain injury: A comparison of two tasks. *Journal of Medical Speech-Language Pathology, 8*, 15–25.

Takakuwa, K. M., Rubashkin, N., & Herzig, K. E. (2004). *What I learned in medical school: Personal stories of young doctors.* Berkeley: University of California Press.

Tedlock, B. (2000). Ethnography and ethnographic representation. In N. K. Denzin & Y. S. Lincoln (Eds.), *Handbook of qualitative research* (pp. 455–486). Thousand Oaks, CA: Sage.

Tedlock, B. (2003). Ethnography and ethnographic representation. In N. K. Denzin & Y. S. Lincoln (Eds.), *Strategies of qualitative inquiry* (2nd ed., pp. 165–213). Thousand Oaks, CA: Sage.

Tharpe, A. M., Rassi, J. A. & Biswas, G. (1995). Problem-Based Learning: An innovative approach to audiology education. *American Journal of Audiology, 4*, 19–25.

Thomas, F. P. (1984). *How to write the story of your life.* Cincinnati, OH: Writer's Digest Books.

Thorne, A., & McLean, K. C. (2003). Telling traumatic events in adolescence: A study of master narrative positioning. In R. Fivush & C. A. Haden (Eds.), *Connecting culture and memory: The development of an autobiographical self* (pp. 169–186). Mahwah, NJ: Lawrence Erlbaum.

Tierney, W. G. (2003). Undaunted courage: Life history and the postmodern challenge. In N. K. Denzin & Y. S. Lincoln (Eds.), *Strategies of qualitative inquiry* (2nd ed., pp. 537-555). Thousand Oaks, CA: Sage.

Todd, L. (1999). Node-link mapping as an alternative to therapeutic writing. *Dissertation Abstracts International, 59*(8-B), 567.

Tompkins, C. A. (1995). *Right hemisphere communication disorders: Theory and management.* San Diego, CA: Singular.

Trautman, L. S., Healey, E. C., & Brown, T. A. (1999). A further analysis of narrative skills of children who stutter. *Journal of Communication Disorders, 32,* 297-315.

Treadway. D. C. (2004). *Intimacy, change, and other therapeutic mysteries: Stories of clinicians and clients.* New York: Guilford Press.

Trupe, E., & Hillis, A. (1985). Paucity vs. verbosity: Another analysis of right hemisphere communication deficits. In R. Brookshire (Ed.), *Clinical aphasiology* (p. 15) Minneapolis, MN: BRK.

Ulatowska, H. K., Allard, L., Reyes, B. A., Ford, J., & Chapman, S. B. (1992). Conversational discourse in aphasia. *Aphasiology, 6,* 325-331.

Ulatowska, H. K., & Bond, S. A. (1983). Aphasia: Discourse considerations. *Topics in Language Disorders, 3,* 21-34.

Ulatowska, H. K., Doyel, A. W., Stern, R. F., & Haynes, S. M. (1983). Production of procedural discourse in aphasia. *Brain and Language, 18,* 315-341.

Ulatowska, H. K., North, A. J., & Macaluso-Haynes, S. (1981). Production of narrative and procedural discourse in aphasia. *Brain and Language, 13,* 345-371.

Ulatowska, H. K., Wertz, R. T., Chapman, S. B., Hill, C. L., Thompson, J. L., Keebler, M. W., et al. (2001). Interpretation of fables and proverbs by African Americans with and without aphasia. *American Journal of Speech-Language Pathology, 10,* 40-50.

van Dulmen, S., & van den Brink-Muinen, A. (2004). Patients' preferences and experiences in handling emotions: A study on communication sequences in primary care medical visits. *Patient Education and Counseling, 55,* 149-152.

Vickers, M. H. (2003). Expectations of consistency in organizational life: Stories of inconsistency from people with unseen chronic illness. *Employee Responsibilities and Rights Journal, 15,* 85-98.

Voneche, J. (2001). Identity and narrative in Piaget's autobiographies. In J. Brockmeier & D. Carbaugh (Eds.), *Narrative and identity: Studies in autobiography, self and culture.* Philadelphia: John Benjamin.

Wagner, C. R., Nettelbladt, U., & Sahlen, B., & Nilholm, B. (2000). Conversation versus narration in pre-school children with language impairment. *International Journal of Language & Communication Disorders, 35,* 83-93.

Walker, K. L., & Dickson, F. C. (2004). An exploration of illness-related narratives in marriage: The identification of illness-identity scripts. *Journal of Social and Personal Relationships, 21,* 521-544.

Waxman, D. (2005). Don't just do something, stand there. *Families, Systems, & Health, 23,* 362-363.

Wear, D., & Aultman, J. M. (2005). The limits of narrative: Medical student resistance to confronting inequality and oppression in literature and beyond. *Medical Education, 39,* 1056-1065.

Weber, K. (2006). *Triangle.* New York: Farrar, Strauss, & Giroux.

Weingarten, K., & Weingarten Worthen, M. E. (1999). A narrative approach to understanding the illness experiences of a mother and daughter. In R. P. Marinellil & A. E. Dell Orto (Eds.), *The psychological and social impact of disability* (pp. 116-133). New York: Springer.

Weir, W. (2005, November 14). Combat inspires soldiers to pick up a pen. *Miami Herald,* p. E1.

Wells, T., Falk S., & Dieppe, P. (2004). The patients' written word: A simple communication aid. *Patient Education and Counseling, 54,* 197-200.

West, C. (1984). When the doctor is a "lady": Power, status, and gender in physician-patient encounters. *Symbolic Interaction, 7,* 87-106.

West, R. (2005). Time for a change: Putting the Transtheoretical (Stages of Change) model to rest. *Addiction, 100,* 1036-1039.

Whelan, K. K., Huber, J., Rose, C., Davies, A., & Clandinin, D. J. (2001). Telling and retelling our stories on the professional knowledge landscape. *Teachers and Teaching: Theory and Practice, 7,* 143-156.

White, H. (1981). The value of narrativity in the representation of reality. In W. J. T. Mitchell (Ed.), *On narrative* (pp. 5-27). Chicago: University of Chicago Press.

Widdershoven, G. A. M., & Smits, M. J. (1996). Ethics and narratives. In R. Josselson (Ed), *Narrative study of lives* (Vol. 4, pp. 275-287). Thousand Oaks, CA: Sage.

Wilkinson, R. (2004). Reflecting on talk in speech and language therapy: Some contributions using conversation analysis. *International Journal of Language & Communication Disorders, 39,* 497-503.

Woike, B. A. (1995). Most-memorable experiences: Evidence for a link between implicit and explicit motives and social cognitive processes in everyday life. *Journal of Personality and Social Psychology, 68,* 1081-1091.

World Health Organization. (2001). *International classification of functioning, disability, and health* (ICF). Geneva: Author.

Wright-St. Clair, V. (2003). Story making and storytelling: Making sense of living with multiple sclerosis. *Journal of Occupational Science, 10,* 46-51.

Yorkston, K. M., & Beukelman, D. (1980). An analysis of connected speech samples of aphasic and normal speakers. *Journal of Speech and Hearing Disorders*, *45*, 27–36.

Young, K., & Saver, J. L. (2001). The neurology of narrative. *SubStance*, *30*, 72–84.

Youse, K. M., & Coelho, C. A. (2005). Working memory and discourse production abilities following traumatic brain injury. *Brain Injury*, *19*, 1001–1009.

Index